Developing the Wise Doctor

Developing the Wise Doctor

A resource for trainers and trainees in MMC

Della Fish
Professor (postgraduate studies)
School of Health Science, University of Wales, Swansea

Linda de Cossart
Consultant Vascular and General Surgeon
Countess of Chester NHS Foundation Trust and Council Member,
The Royal College of Surgeons of England

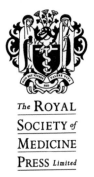

The ROYAL
SOCIETY of
MEDICINE
PRESS Limited

Published in Great Britain in 2011 by
Hodder Arnold, an imprint of Hodder Education, an Hachette UK company,
338 Euston Road, London NW1 3BH

www.hodderarnold.com

First published by The Royal Society of Medicine Press Ltd, 1 Wimpole Street, London W1G 0AE, UK
The logo of The Royal Society of Medicine is a registered trade mark, which it has licensed to Hodder Arnold.

Hachette UK's policy is to use papers that are natural, renewable and recyclable products and made from wood
grown in sustainable forests. The logging and manufacturing processes are expected to conform to the
environmental regulations of the country of origin.

Whilst the advice and information in this book are believed to be true and accurate at the date of going to press,
neither the author[s] nor the publisher can accept any legal responsibility or liability for any errors or omissions
that may be made. In particular, (but without limiting the generality of the preceding disclaimer) every effort has
been made to check drug dosages; however it is still possible that errors have been missed. Furthermore, dosage
schedules are constantly being revised and new side-effects recognized. For these reasons the reader is strongly
urged to consult the drug companies' printed instructions before administering any of the drugs recommended in
this book.

British Library Cataloguing in Publication Data
A catalogue record for this book is available from the British Library

Library of Congress Cataloging-in-Publication Data
A catalog record for this book is available from the Library of Congress

ISBN-13 9781853156182

1 2 3 4 5 6 7 8 9 10

Typeset by Phoenix Photosetting
Printed and bound in the UK by Bell & Bain

What do you think about this book? Or any other Hodder Arnold title?
Please visit our website: www.hodderarnold.com

Contents

Figures, tables and resources

FIGURES

TABLES

RESOURCES

Glossary

A & E	Accident and Emergency
C-bD	Case-based Discussion
Cons.	Consultant
CT scan	Computerized tomography scan
DOPS	Direct Observation of Procedural Skills
DVDs	Digital video disc
DVT	Deep vein thrombosis
F1 doctor	Foundation Year 1 doctor
F2 doctor	Foundation Year 2 doctor
GMC	General Medical Council
GPPS	The General Professional Practice of Surgery
MDT	Multi-Disciplinary Team
METB	Medical Education and Training Board
MiniCEX	Mini-Clinical Evaluation Exercise
MMC	Modernising Medical Careers
NHS	National Health Service
OCAPs	Orthopaedic Competence Assessment Procedure
OP COMP	Operative Competence
OT	Occupational Therapist
PA view	Professional Artistry view
PAT	Peer-Assessment Tool
PMETB	Postgraduate Medical Education and Training Board
TA	Triggered Assessment
TR view	Technical Rational view
RITA	Record of In-Training Assessment
RCP	Royal College of Physicians
SpR	Specialist Registrar
UK	United Kingdom

Acknowledgements

Formal thanks are due to the Picasso Administration for permission to use and reproduce Picasso's painting *Science and Charity* on both the cover of this book and in Chapter 9.

We are particularly grateful to Professor Alastair Vincent Campbell (Professor in Medical Ethics), Yong Loo Lin School of Medicine, Singapore, for his kind permission to use in our Chapter 9 significant amounts of text and ideas from his classic book *Moderated Love,* and for the great encouragement he gave us in seeing our work as a useful follow-up to his.

We have also been delighted to receive from Kathryn Montgomery encouragement and permission to quote from her important new book *How Doctors Think,* which resonates with both this book and our earlier writing.

We note with thanks the permission of the Open University Press to use some small parts of Della Fish's and Colin Coles' *Medical Education: Developing a Curriculum for Practice,* and yet again record appreciative thanks for the oral and written ideas of Professor Michael Golby of Exeter University, as acknowledged in our text. We also thank Dr Pam Shaw of Kent, Surrey and Sussex Postgraduate Deanery for highlighting the importance of developing what lies at the periphery of one's vision.

Jo Richardson (Head of Medical Imaging at The Countess of Chester NHS Foundation Trust) and her colleague Jenni Collins created for us, as a private commission, the exact illustration we wanted for the heuristic for Chapter 10, which we think brings this entire book together. We thank them for their patience, persistence and expertise.

We also thank all our colleagues in medical practice and medical education who have helped us in many ways. Amongst these we particularly acknowledge the following:

- medical and surgical practitioners in hospital Trusts (particularly The Countess of Chester NHS Foundation Trust, and other Trusts in Merseyside and the South of England) whose practice has inspired our thinking, whose response to our ideas has been supportive and challenging, and who have helped us see how to create practical resources for use in the clinical setting
- our educational colleagues and all the committed surgeon and physician educators in Kent, Surrey and Sussex Deanery, and the Deaneries of Mersey and Wessex, who have sustained and encouraged us in the struggle to clarify and articulate what is involved in the practice of medical education and its role in the clinical setting
- Jean Douglas and Evelyn Usher, whose highly focused proof-reading has saved us from numerous errors, has enabled us to send to the Press a text that expressed our ideas clearly, and who bear no responsibility for any remaining mistakes
- all those at the RSM Press who have helped this publication on its way into the world and for making the process smooth and enjoyable, especially Laura Compton and Nathan Harris for their determination to get the cover as we really wanted it, and Hannah Wessely, who oversaw the entire project and who, despite some changes of plan on our part, never ceased to be supportive.

It should be noted that the ideas contained in this publication are our own and are not necessarily shared by any institutions for which we work.

Foreword

The education and training of our medical force is changing as fast as the practice of medicine itself. It is a pleasure to be associated with this publication that is bringing together several exciting elements in medical education. They include a critical, evidence-based approach, an understanding of the obligations of the trainee, the best use of limited time and clear underpinning principles of medical professionalism. There has been much good about the overarching principles of Modernising Medical Careers, but it is important that these are not lost in a quest to deliver a 'one size fits all' national process that stifles innovation. Innovations that are truly worthwhile should encourage the brightest and best to be stretched whilst bringing on those who learn more slowly.

This publication reminds us that medical education is important, it is a contract between trainee and trainer, it must adhere to sound and critical evidence and it should enhance, not diminish, the professional principles that underpin our care for patients. Finally it should be fun! The authors are to be congratulated for letting these key principles shine through, and I welcome the promise of these themes being extended in future publications.

Professor Ian Gilmore
President, Royal College of Physicians
May 2007

Introduction

We believe that Postgraduate Medical Education in the UK has reached a key defining moment in terms of the quality of its educational ideas and processes.

Modernising Medical Careers (MMC: the government's project to reshape the medical profession) set out to place firmly *in the clinical setting* not only the teaching, but also the assessment and the recording of the progress of postgraduate doctors. This was itself an important landmark. But it brought with it a rather basic and somewhat uncritical approach to the postgraduate education of practising doctors. This is perhaps partly because of its aim to be simple enough for every clinical supervisor and supervisee to operate quickly during the busyness of practice without the need for extensive and expensive educational help and support. But it is also partly because it has borrowed assessment materials from other cultures, professions and arenas rather than starting by both analysing the nature of clinical practice as experienced by working doctors in the UK, and defining the values and principles that underpin good professional postgraduate education everywhere.

The result, we believe, has been an overwhelming sameness – both in learners' assessment processes through the Foundation and now into Speciality Training (where the same 'Tools of the Trade' continue to be used), and in the results of all this, which do not seem to us to be good at differentiating and celebrating the range of talent that postgraduate doctors bring to and develop within medical practice.

It seems to us that it is now time to attune the education of doctors more finely, in order to engage them in enjoying the exploration of their practice and to provide challenging new ways of thinking about it, so that they develop not only their practical skills but also the vital understanding that determines how, when, why and where those skills should be employed. In doing so, we have borne in mind the pressures of time and the extreme demands of clinical practice, and have designed what we offer so that it is achievable within this climate.

1

OUR AIMS

In short, we seek in this book to develop on from the achievements of MMC. We thus highlight the importance of making explicit the invisible elements of medical practice, of developing these and of assessing them. To this end, we offer a wide range of ideas, materials and resources, together with a language in which to discuss them, that will enrich the curriculum for postgraduate medical education in the clinical setting.

Our aim is to foster exploration of practice and enrich understanding. We seek to do so by indicating ideals to reach for, offering ideas to extend understanding, and providing activities to challenge both the practice doctors engage in and the theories that lie behind it. We thereby hope to encourage well-supported but open-ended development that allows the best doctors to fly, the more steady to grow proportionately and the more needy to review, recover and remediate their difficulties – and all of these to demonstrate and record the evidence as appropriate.

We also wish to open this entire enterprise (both our particular contribution and the wider endeavour of current postgraduate medical education) to a greater criticality in which theory is used to challenge practice and practice is brought up to critique theory. Criticality is, after all, one important and defining characteristic of any postgraduate education.

We cannot emphasize too strongly, however, that the vehicle for such educational development, is discussion – reflective discussion with peers, but also with supervisors, seniors and experts in other professions – and, in respect of some events in their practice, also some writing (the very process of which often produces even deeper understanding). New postgraduate doctors are emerging from secondary and undergraduate education with experience of the importance of both speaking and writing as key educational processes. But their teachers are less secure in these.

The discussion we refer to here is, as a two-way process, well characterized by the term 'professional conversation'. This marks a key characteristic of our approach. We believe that postgraduate doctors can equip themselves with much of the information that seniors in the past used to 'deliver' to them, and instead can use the small opportunities with those seniors and other experts to move beyond the passive learner mode and explore, consider, put into their own words, challenge, critique, and embed a better understood and more robust version of them within their own experience and understanding. This means that teachers and learners need to have to hand a range of resources that will guide the work that learners might do in order to prepare for and gain from a deeper discussion with their teachers. We have sought to provide such resources, a language in which to explore them and some enjoyable ways of remembering the important elements.

THE STRUCTURE OF THE BOOK

To this end, the book falls into two parts. The first part shows that many of the national postgraduate medical curricula currently available focus on the more visible and easily identified aspects of medical practice. It explains how our ideas fit with and extend this current postgraduate medical education, and it discusses in depth how teachers and learners in the clinical setting might use the resources we offer in Part Two.

This second part offers a range of ideas, resources and language for teachers and learners to use to explore what we refer to as the invisible elements of practice. This is followed by an Appendix that offers an overview of what an enriched curriculum might attend to and shows how the ideas we offer can extend and deepen the education of doctors as well as providing a means of assessment that does justice to the complexity of medical practice.

THE READERSHIP OF THIS BOOK

We address the ideas in this book to all postgraduate doctors who teach and learn in the clinical setting, and all those who support them (for example, educationists and managers who need to understand better what medical education is about).

This book takes its examples from teaching and learning in Secondary Care, but is equally relevant to General Practitioners, who in any case will all have had some experience in hospital-based medicine as part of the Foundation Programme and in their specialty education and training programme.

We introduce a number of themes, many of which may be new to both teachers and learners who practice medicine, and some of which we intend to treat in greater detail in publications to come.

AND FINALLY ...

We believe that learning and teaching are and should be fun. Many people tell us that that it is how it used to be. In working with considerable numbers of doctors to develop and refine our ideas, we (and we think they too) have daily rediscovered that deeply pleasurable element.

Our 'enrichment curriculum' is thus concerned with helping doctors achieve greater understanding and better-supported practice in both medicine and medical education, and is also dedicated to re-instituting the enjoyment that comes from learners and teachers challenging themselves and each other.

We invite readers to use and critique this book in the belief that educational ideas, if used with proper criticality, will always enhance the thinking of teachers and learners and can always be developed and refined.

Part One

Postgraduate medicine and medical education: Current 'dis-ease' and possible cure

1

Learning in clinical practice: Two visions for the future

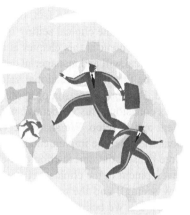

INTRODUCTION

The Foundation Programme in the UK for doctors in their first two years of post-graduate training is now fully established. Phased in from 2004 onwards, it has set out to revolutionize the experiences of those who are known as Foundation Year 1 (F1) and Foundation Year 2 (F2) doctors. It has also had a considerable effect upon those who teach these new doctors and it has substantially influenced the specialty training curricula now being drafted for the new run-through grades that follow the Foundation years.

The national policy for Modernising Medical Careers (MMC) contains a vision of postgraduate medical education that has spawned both the Foundation pro-gramme and the new regulatory body, the Postgraduate Medical Education and Training Board (PMETB), which itself seems set soon to be truncated to METB and to cover undergraduate courses also. The quality and extent of MMC's edu-cational vision is to be found crystallized in the Foundation curriculum. We have therefore focused much of the detailed analysis that follows on that concrete example, which is representative of the official overall view of education for doc-tors in the 21st century.

We, like many, have already critiqued the early development of MMC and of the Foundation curriculum in another publication, (see Fish and Coles, 2005, Chapter 1). However, we note with some sadness that although it will be repub-lished in 2007, it will appear in a redrafted but not a reconceived version. It there-fore appears that the vision enshrined in the Foundation curriculum seems set to underpin and shape the future education of doctors in the UK for the early decades of the 21st century.

We doubt that in its present form it is equal to this task, because it lacks a depth of resource to support learners and provides few educational strategies to support properly to either. For example, because the assessors change each time an assessment form is used, learners are not easily helped to see how they are actually progressing day by day.

Assessment will never be a scientific and objective activity. It must be fair – but this is not the same as 'objective'. Interpretation is an unavoidable and important element in assessment. This means that multiple perspectives need to be collected about a learner and 'the soundness of the assessment is ... related to the rigour with which those multiple perspectives are collected, recorded, interpreted and utilized. But this should not be a substitute for the main teacher having a clear and well documented understanding of the learner's progress' (Fish and Coles, 2005, p. 171).

'Tools of the Trade' use multiple assessors, and thus fulfil the requirements of multiple perspectives. But they fail to attend to the rigour and interpretation with which those perspectives are collected. In addition, they fail to offer the learner and main teacher a sense of continuity in respect of the learner's developing achievements.

Assessment is concerned with 'demonstrating how well, and in what ways, a learner has profited from the learning opportunities provided, and with recording these achievements and the learner's educational progress' (de Cossart and Fish, 2005, p. 98). The final goal of all assessment processes should be to equip the learner to become good at self-assessment.

The 'Tools of the Trade' are clearly not designed to place a priority on these educational intentions. Rather, they are designed to imbue in trainees a set of skills that are presented as 'generic' to all medicine, and which the curriculum implies are therefore the key to what new doctors should be learning. This is why the curriculum is described as 'competency-based'. However, it is principles, not skills, that are generic. Thus, as we shall now show, competence (a holistic understanding of practice and an all-round ability to carry it out) is arguably a better goal for the Foundation curriculum than competencies (a series of discrete skills that are learnt and assessed separately).

Generic skills and the myth of measurement

If skills were 'generic' (implying that they are identical across all contexts) *then* to learn skills in one context would be sufficient to ensure that they could be fully and appropriately used in all others. Were this the case, the learning of skills on a small scale would provide all that was needed to guarantee successful professional practice. However, this conveniently ignores the significance of the context. Once criticality is brought to bear on this notion, it takes very little thought to recognize that skills need to be adapted significantly from context to context, and that they are best adapted on a *principled* basis. In other words, what matter at least as much as skills are the *principles* that guide the adaptation of skills.

Competencies, which are presented as the basis of the Foundation curriculum, are concerned only with visible behaviour and its measurement. This view of professional work overlooks the subtleties of sensitivity, imagination, wisdom, standard rather than a base-level one (as identified by the Foundation curriculum). This is because we share with the authors of the Royal College of Physicians' (RCP's) report on *Doctors in Society: Medical Professionalism in a Changing World*, the view that 'doctors have a perpetual commitment to the continuous improvement of their practice through continuous professional development (p. 21), and because we too want to set a higher standard even than 'competence'. We too believe that it is time to stress the idea of working once again towards *excellence* and see this as 'the possession of abilities to an eminent or meritorious degree' (RCP, 2005, p. 17).

We believe that doctors should be exploring and seeking to develop their own practice in the light of these elements and that they should use the standard to be achieved as their ultimate target.

In the right-hand column of Table 1.1 we have indicated methods for assessing doctors' abilities to recognize and utilize these elements. We have also indicated to what extent the 'Tools of the Trade' provide for this kind of assessment, and we have commented on the limited extent to which they provide evidence of the standard of individual doctor's achievements.

In looking at this table, it will quickly become clear that the assessment processes (the tick-box approach to recording), provide no detailed means of developing, assessing and giving evidence of achievement in any of the elements. Quite simply, the forms for 'Tools of the Trade', do little more than record that a discussion or observation has taken place. The quality of the learner's achievements is offered on a scale that leads to gross generalization, and the end-result is to make all learners look alike.

By contrast, we are arguing for learning and assessment in postgraduate medicine to be based on a far more detailed and rich understanding of clinical practice. We believe that these elements are all best explored in the light of a patient case or the engagement with a medical procedure. This is why we think that DOPs and C-bD are the two assessment tools that can be built upon. We would particularly wish to provide opportunities for spoken and written reflection that would take learners beyond the DOPs and C-bD forms to look at the less visible elements of the simple practice that has been recorded on those forms, and many of the following chapters offer ways of doing this.

Whose responsibility is it to take this vision on?

The basis of our motivation in offering this book is a profound belief that those working in the clinical setting can begin to put this enrichment process into practice now, without additional preparation beyond what we offer here. We have provided for teachers and learners at all levels in postgraduate medicine a full account of the teaching strategies needed, the ideas to explore and the resources to use in relation to clinical practice in order to think about it more deeply. We are convinced that in using critically what we offer here to explore these more challenging aspects of practice (alongside the national curricula requirements), teachers and learners will develop new clinical and educational understanding.

- It does not focus on the extent to which the doctor is a rounded professional, nor on how well they collaborate with patients and other colleagues.
- Above all, it emphasizes only their technical accountability.

Clearly, this is a very negative view of what is happening and a pessimistic appraisal of the Foundation Programme's current achievements. Our view is that the current philosophy of MMC is based upon the kind of thinking that politicians and managers engage in, but that doctors in postgraduate medical education and their patients deserve their curricula to be based upon the most soundly logical educational thinking and a full understanding of the complexities of clinical practice. In the following section, we therefore illustrate what an analysis of medical practice suggests that young doctors need to learn and to demonstrate in the assessment of their practice, and we look at how far the 'Tools of the Trade' assist with this.

ENRICHING THE VISION: REDIRECTING MEDICAL EDUCATION TO DEVELOP WISE PRACTICE

So what might extend and enrich this vision?

Those aspects that are listed above as currently missing from the content sections of the curriculum and its assessment processes are by and large not found on the visible face of medical practice. In analysing the practice of working doctors, we have identified nine elements of practice (seven main points and two subcategories) that seem to us to characterize their complex and lived experience, and which need to be attended to by all postgraduate medical curricula. These are:

1a. The significance of context in understanding the patient case and coming to crucial decisions related to medical practice

1b. The importance of the doctor's personal qualities as contributing to the interpretation of the context (a subsection of the point above)

2. The fundamental influence of the doctor's values in shaping the response to all that is met in medical practice

3a. The forms of knowledge that the doctor uses in practice

3b. The technical processes, procedures and skills that the doctor uses in practice (a subsection of the point above)

4. The clinical thinking that the doctor engages in

5. The professional judgements that the doctor reaches

6. The ability to establish a sound therapeutic relationship with the patient and to engage in holistic medicine

7. The ability to work reflectively in the social and clinical complexities of practice and continue to extend and deepen a holistic version of practice.

We present these elements of clinical practice in Table 1.1. For each element we have, in the left-hand column, offered a more detailed definition and an indication of the standard to be achieved at the highest level. This is an aspirational

- self-knowledge and the ability of a professional to attend to their own professional development
- the ability to influence key decisions at the level of policy and the capacity to take an active role in the development of the profession itself.

In the light of this analysis, the following section summarizes the key elements of the MMC's current vision for medical education, and pinpoints the aspects of clinical practice that are not attended to at all. The final section will then introduce an enriched version of this vision that prepares the way for the rest of the book.

THE MISREPRESENTATION OF MEDICAL PRACTICE AND THE MISDIRECTION OF MEDICAL EDUCATION

We believe that it becomes clear from our analysis that the Foundation curriculum's intentions are managerial rather than educational. They are about establishing national control over medical education rather than educating doctors to the highest possible level. We see national policy for medicine as seduced by the value of the superficial and simplistic, and by the idea that what is measurable is inevitably significant. We see the myth of generic skills promulgated in order to minimize doctors' educational needs and economize on educational resources. In short, we fear that in emphasizing only the visible and easily understood elements of practice, current requirements for postgraduate medicine misrepresent medical practice and misdirect medical education.

The vision of the Foundation curriculum

We characterize this educationally impoverished vision as follows (see also de Cossart and Fish, 2005, p. 100):

- It ignores the significance of context in learning to practise medicine and seems to assume that assessment can be context-neutral.
- It is not interested in requiring doctors to be aware of and confront their own attitudes, values, assumptions, beliefs and personal theories that drive their actions and are thus part of the context of their practice.
- It treats 'professionalism' as if it were a simple matter of good self-presentation and of talking nicely to patients.
- It ignores the thinking and the knowledge that lie behind the skills and how, in real practice, doctors adapt their knowledge and improvise their skill.
- It does not make central the moral and ethical dimensions of medical practice.
- It offers no way of developing or assessing professional judgement.
- It shows little interest in teaching doctors to establish sound and therapeutic relationships with patients.

judgement and moral awareness that are the mark of a wise doctor. The Western world has an overriding obsession with measurement (see Broadfoot, 1996). But this is at the cost of treating teaching and learning in terms of an industrial trans-action, where what is important is what will conduce to the efficient and cheap delivery of a product – both healthcare and the education for healthcare. Further, the myth of measurement (that it appears to render assessment clear-cut and objective, scientific and absolute), merely covers up the processes of judgement that inevitably underpin such 'measurement'. And this in turn means that the bases of such judgements are not transparent, not public, and not able to be cri-tiqued or developed.

Another 'selling point' of competencies is that they are simple to derive in the first place and also to teach, learn and assess. But this too hides a number of myths. For example, one key problem is that there is no end to the breaking down of skills into finer and finer detail. We have listed other problems elsewhere (de Cossart and Fish, 2005).

By contrast, *competence* is concerned with a holistic notion of professional practice, and the assessment of this is based upon judgements of quality, the bases of which are made explicit. It is concerned with seeing the necessary skills of pro-fessional practice in a wider context, which takes account of the essence, core and complexity of what is really involved in being a professional. A competence-based approach to practice recognizes that professionals exercise judgement and wisdom that goes beyond protocols. They work in creative ways that may draw upon skills but that develop, adapt and improvise them. The work of Carr (1993) provides details of how and why people have muddled these two concepts.

The competence approach values the following (de Cossart and Fish, 2005, pp. 109–10):

- professional practice as involving open capacities that cannot be mastered
- professional judgement and its complexity (the ability to choose between competing priorities, values, actions, interpretations)
- the complex and uncertain nature of day-to-day practice
- professionals' moral responsibility to vulnerable patients/clients and to colleagues, and, in addition, professional answerability in respect of their technical proficiency
- the ability to utilize general knowledge, thinking and doing (which includes skills, but also far more), so that they are shaped to the specific and particular individual needs of patients
- the development of a (personal) principled base from which to practise as a professional
- an understanding of the importance of values and self-knowledge
- the need to attend to the moral and ethical dimensions of practice
- an understanding of the wider issues of professionalism and the responsibilities of being a member of a profession
- the use of a range of skills and of the importance of choosing rationally between them

3b. Technical processes and procedures carried out by the practitioner (focus on procedural knowledge)

(i) Definition
The ability to carry out satisfactorily all key procedures required within clinical practice, including technical and operative competence as appropriate to the specialty

(ii) Standard
The ability to set up and carry out procedures to a high level of practice such that close supervision is no longer necessary

DOPS and MiniCEX
Triggered Assessment (TA)/Operative Competence (OP COMP), and Orthopaedic Competence Assessment Procedure (OCAPs) (in the surgical specialty curricula)

DOPS, OP COMP and OCAPs give useful formative experience, but do not aim to give summative evidence to satisfy the standard

TA is a summative assessment that if performed rigorously attends to the standard

4. Clinical thinking that the practitioner engages in

(i) Definition
The ability to engage successfully in:
- framing the case
- clinical reasoning
- clinical solutions
- deliberation
- practical wisdom
- using personal professional judgement

(ii) Standard
The ability to be focused and fluent about each given case with respect to all the aspects listed above

CASE-BASED DISCUSSION

C-bD offers a truncated and generalized version of the thinking that has happened, because it does not require a rigorous unearthing of all the implicit and tacit thinking that has occurred.

23

Table 1.1 continued

Element of practice to be learnt and assessed, and standard to be aimed for	Assessment tool/method and quality of evidence available
5. The ability to formulate sound professional judgements and to engage in wise practice	
(i) Definition **The ability to select from a range of possible judgements a high quality professional judgement**	**There is no means of assessing this in depth**
(ii) Standard *Consistency of sound professional judgement that is the best for each individual patient and the capacity to defend/argue for, implement and lead consequent actions*	No reliable evidence of how these judgements are reached (the actions could be the result of either sound clinical thinking or good luck), and there will be no conclusive evidence of which of these is the case.
6. The ability to establish a sound therapeutic relationship with the patient and engage in holistic medical practice	
(i) Definition **A wise doctor is one who can harness consideration of all the elements of practice in the best interests of each patient and establish a restorative and healing relationship with them (irrespective of the ability to cure), which enriches both doctor and patient**	**CASE-BASED DISCUSSION** **Only in respect of the *tone*, which is not documented in the form**
(ii) Standard *Consistency of the therapeutic relationship, meaning that it is established with every patient as far as is possible, and not just with those with whom it is easy to work*	The 'tone' of the case discussed in C-bD is rarely considered, and can be 'put on' rather than genuine. Unless the doctor is asked to discuss the therapeutic relationship, it can only be glimpsed occasionally in everyday practice

7. The ability to work reflectively in the socially and clinically complex practice setting and extend and deepen a holistic vision of clinical practice

(i) Definition
The ability to reflect during practice as well as afterwards, and to notice and be able to explore the ever wider and deeper aspects of practice (both the social and the clinical) that become evident with increasing experience.

(ii) Standard
Consistency of overall development

REQUIRED IN THE PORTFOLIO
(but no indication of how it can be assessed)

No criteria have been developed for how to assess the portfolio, and thus there is no concrete evidence for either the learner or future teachers of whether or not a learner's progress is sound and consistent

We therefore invite readers, whilst responding as required to national demands, at the same time to explore critically what we offer in the following pages and to try out some of the ideas and the resources that we provide.

FURTHER READING

Broadfoot P (1996) 'Educational assessment: the myth of measurement'. (Inaugural Lecture given at the University of Bristol on 25 October 1993). In: Woods P, ed. *Contemporary Issues on Teaching and Learning.* London: Routledge/Open University: 203–33.

de Cossart L, Fish, D (2005) *Cultivating a Thinking Surgeon: New Perspectives on Clinical Teaching, Learning and Assessment.* Shrewsbury: tfm Publications.

de Cossart L, Fish D (2006) Thinking outside the (tick) box: rescuing professionalism and professional judgement. *Med Educ* **40**: 403–5.

Fish D, Coles C (2005) *Medical Education: Developing a Curriculum for Practice.* Maidenhead: Open University Press.

2

Wise practice for better patient care: Introducing 'the invisibles' and the heuristics

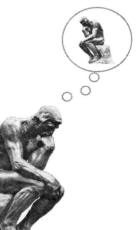

INTRODUCTION

We argued in Chapter 1 that the goals of the Foundation curriculum, and of those specialty specific curricula that are modelled on it, are not concerned with establishing a quality education for doctors. An analysis of these goals suggests that the elements to be learnt and in which doctors will be assessed have been chosen in order to ensure a utilitarian and economic approach to educating postgraduate doctors and because they are visible and easily quantifiable. The outcomes of MMC in its current form will produce efficient technicians who will comply with the controlling demands of managers.

We have argued that this curriculum is not based upon an accurate account of the character of medical practice, and thus short-changes patients. We have offered nine elements of practice that we believe postgraduate medical education should include, and have shown in Table 1.1 that the Foundation programme attends in detail to only one of these. In designing ways of enriching this curriculum, we have been concerned to establish a higher-quality goal for postgraduate doctors, namely that of becoming a wise practitioner. We believe that this is what patients deserve.

In this chapter, there are four sections. Firstly, we explain how we have developed our ideas. Secondly, we introduce and offer an overview of what we have come to call 'the invisibles' and how they can enrich the curriculum and equip doctors to provide documented evidence of their achievements and progress. We then show how the invisibles relate to a set of heuristics (or prompts) to help learners to remember the invisibles in the clinical setting. Finally, we offer some thoughts about the relationship of the invisibles with the 'Tools of the Trade', and show how they complement and enrich these assessment processes. A detailed exploration of each of these enriching elements is then to be found, chapter by chapter, in Part Two of this book.

THE DEVELOPMENT OF OUR IDEAS

The most significant point that we wish to make about how we developed these ideas is that they emerged from an extensive analysis of the clinical practice of a number of doctors. This has also been underpinned by an exploration of what others have published about the nature of medical practice. The detail of much of this we have already made public in Fish and Coles (2005, Chapters 4 and 5).

We have also been privileged both individually and together to engage in a wide number of educational activities that have caused us to distil and crystallize our thinking and how to articulate it. The following are key examples.

The educational development activities we have engaged in include the writing of two national curricula. One of these, the curriculum for the early years of surgical training – known as The General Professional Practice of Surgery (GPPS) – on which we worked together, has now been subsumed into the new Intercollegiate Surgical Curriculum. The other, the curriculum for Surgical Care Practitioners, emerged from a national group chaired by Linda de Cossart and was published by the Department of Health in 2005. We also engaged in writing and publishing two books in 2005, which are focused on medical education (de Cossart and Fish, 2005; Fish and Coles, 2005).

We have used and developed our ideas both with consultant teachers and with doctors in training, at a variety of levels across a number of seminars and seminar series in the last three years. Programmes in which we have engaged doctors in better understanding their clinical practice by using the invisibles have included:

- five seminars designed to support GPPS in one hospital Trust in Kent, Surrey and Sussex Postgraduate Deanery and in two hospital Trusts in Mersey Deanery
- a range of seminars in Chester designed to explore our ideas with consultants
- in-house teaching of four half-day seminars to surgical trainees
- a 3½ day programme for 53 doctors on the 2005–06 Early Years of Surgical Training Year 1, in Mersey Deanery; and a similar programme for 15 trainees for 2006–07
- two programmes of four half-days each for F2s in Chester
- three programmes of seven half-day sessions for doctors and non-medical practitioners who were learning the role of First Assistant
- major contributions to two masters degree pathways for Teaching and Learning in the clinical setting that were designed for doctors and are offered in two different Deaneries
- a wide range of day seminars over the last three years for Cardiff University School of Healthcare Studies' Postgraduate and Continuing Education Unit
- an invitation day seminar for consultants and senior educators.

We are therefore indebted to a huge number of doctors and educators (too numerous to name) for helping us to explore and refine the following ideas.

INTRODUCING 'THE INVISIBLES', AND HOW THEY CAN ENRICH THE CURRICULUM

We came only gradually to use the term 'the invisibles' to describe the nine elements of practice referred to in Chapter 1. The following explains how this came about.

The invisibles

Eight of the nine elements of practice that we identified in Table 1.1 in Chapter 1 are not immediately visible to an observer of practice (the exception being the technical processes and procedures carried out by the practitioner).

It is vitally important in education for professional practice to unearth knowledge and make it explicit, because this is the major way of developing and refining it. It is almost universally recognized that this is a form of reflecting on practice and that such reflection frequently takes a narrative form and shape.

We believe that the DOPS and C-bD forms require learners to begin to reflect on the stories associated with their patient cases or on their engagement in clinical procedures, but that, ironically, at the same time, the tick-box approach stifles the real potential of this. We are seeking to enrich this part of the learning and assessment process by highlighting the key invisibles of medical practice and offering resources that enable doctors to reflect upon them in detail, so that their development of understanding is recorded in writing and can be placed in the learning portfolio alongside the visible elements recorded on the forms.

The term 'tacit' has been a traditional way of referring to these elements of practice, but we believe that this is not accurate. The following explains why we refer to them instead as the invisibles of practice.

Explicit, implicit and tacit knowledge

Those philosophers who are experts in studying the nature of knowledge recognize three categories of knowledge: the explicit, the implicit and the tacit.

It is our contention that both the implicit and the tacit elements of practice (both of which are invisible) need to be explicated as a key part of postgraduate medical education. But we acknowledge, with Schön (1987a), that by no means all the tacit can be unearthed in this way because some lies too deep for us ever to become conscious of it. We therefore use the term 'the invisibles' to refer to the implicit knowledge that lies beneath the surface of practice together with that amount of the tacit that can be brought back to the surface by the practitioner. The following explains this in more detail.

Explicit knowledge is, of course that which is publicly documented and thus structured, or as Eraut calls it, 'codified' (Eraut and du Boulay, 2000). It is that which practitioners state clearly and often, and which is therefore consciously at the front of their minds. This can include facts, methods, interpretations, conclusions and reports. Explicit knowledge is in the public arena, and is easily identified in these days of the Internet, and the public has total access to it. Many healthcare professions have been set on explicating as much of their knowledge base as possible (especially in relation to good practice in the profession and in the education for that profession) in order to enhance their status. Examples of explicit knowledge in medicine would include textbooks about clinical knowledge, practical processes and procedures, as well as published writing about patient cases, and research. Teachers and learners draw upon explicit knowledge all the time, and both learning and teaching depend upon making knowledge explicit and, by this means, understanding and thus developing and refining it.

By contrast to this, *implicit knowledge* lies just under the surface of the practices of professionals, or can be seen as lying within products, procedures, processes and organizations. In medicine, this is knowledge that is consciously known but not regularly stated and which it is quite possible for doctors to bring to the surface whenever required or prompted to do so. Implicit knowledge is embedded within services, structures, methods and techniques. Some doctors may themselves in the past have merely been trained in or socialized in processes and procedures, and thus have learnt to enact them without unpacking the knowledge and understanding implicit in them. This will make it more difficult for them to share that knowledge now with their learners. But it is imperative that they work to do so, in order to promote the critique and discussion currently needed to prepare these young professionals to explain and defend their knowledge-in-use amongst colleagues and patients, in public and even in courts of law.

Other important forms of implicit knowledge are more personal, and relate to matters such as beliefs, assumptions, and personal theories. To an extent, this is about 'beliefs' rather than 'knowledge', but there is a relationship between these two. Implicit knowledge of this kind can mostly be made explicit with time and thought – but only once its significance has been realized. Again, both teacher and learner need to attend to 'surfacing or re-surfacing' the implicit, but the learner can achieve some of this by inference and without the help of the teacher. But both teacher and learner need to work at this.

Tacit knowledge, by comparison, refers to that knowledge that we do not even recognize that we have. This may be because it is buried inside our thinking and doing, and beneath our experiences and expertise, to a level that renders it unable readily to be retrieved and made conscious or that prevents it from ever being made explicit. In some cases, it may by its very nature be ineffable (inexpressible, unable to be described and characterized), and thus will remain impossible to articulate, except perhaps in metaphorical language.

Much knowledge may always have been (and some will continue to be) tacit in our professional practice, or it may once have been implicit or even explicit, but we no longer see it because routine and custom have put us on autopilot, or simply got in the way of our recognizing it. This, of course, is a great problem for the education of less experienced practitioners. By definition, much of the knowledge that is tacit in senior clinicians is the bedrock of good professional practice and wherever possible needs to be opened up to learners (for reasons explained above), which means that their teachers must struggle to bring back to consciousness as much of it as possible. Indeed, learners need to seek it actively from their seniors in order to lay the foundations for their own practice.

Whilst some practice knowledge will always remain tacit, we believe that much of what is currently 'implicit' in professional practice could be made explicit. We believe that making as much as possible explicit would seriously improve the rigour of teaching professional processes and procedures. Careful reflection on practice and enquiry into it will yield the secret of much of its underlying knowledge, and working with this to turn it into understanding will show us new ways to develop our practice. In many cases, this reflection will take a narrative form. Our development of the invisibles and the resources for exploring clinical practice more fully is precisely to enable doctors (both teachers and learners) to surface, explore and develop this kind of knowledge by using reflection and narrative.

An overview of the invisibles (or: what lies under 'doing' in the clinical setting?)

We would list the invisibles as follows. These take up the main categories of the elements of practice listed in Table 1.1:

1. the significance of context (and the doctor's personal beliefs and assumptions that contribute to the context and shape how s/he sees practice and the practice setting)
2. the professional values the doctor subscribes to
3. the kinds of knowledge the doctor brings to practice
4. the clinical thinking the doctor engages in
5. the professional judgement the doctor exercises
6. the therapeutic relationship the doctor develops with the patient
7. the ability to work reflectively in the socially and clinically complex practice setting and extend and deepen a holistic version of clinical practice

Whilst these elements of practice are not readily visible and thus have not in the past traditionally been explored explicitly as part of medical education, in the current climate of reduced time for postgraduate education, we believe they provide a means to get much more speedily and deeply to the very heart of medical practice. It will then quickly become apparent that the core of medical practice is not technical efficiency that complies with managerial targets. Rather, it involves postgraduate doctors in developing: the wisdom to understand the case, themselves and their role in it more deeply; an awareness of the range of knowledge they are bringing up to it; an ability to weigh the complex and competing priorities involved; the maturity to establish a therapeutic relationship with patients; and the sagacity to come to a wise judgement about treatment, which involves the patient and recognizes the complexity of working and learning in the clinical setting.

Developing the Wise Doctor

The importance of the invisible elements of practice

Thus, we believe that a curriculum that does not ensure that teachers and learners engage with the implicit and the tacit and that focuses its assessment only on visible performance will result in trained technicians who may be technically very skilled but who will not be able to engage in high-quality clinical thinking and sound professional judgement and who therefore will not know when, why, where and how to put their skills to use.

Further, professionals who have not made explicit, developed and refined the professional values upon which their practice is based, will not be so readily articulate in defending their arguments and explaining their reasoning in the many arenas that require this (for example, in talking with patients, colleagues, managers, in courts of law and in career interviews).

The importance of reflection in using the invisibles

We have made the point that reflection (in both spoken and written form) is what gives professional practitioners access to these invisibles and enables both teacher and learner to make explicit both the implicit and, as far as possible, the tacit. The resources we offer in each chapter of Part Two of this book will provide plenty of material to provoke and enhance that reflection.

We have written at length about reflection in de Cossart and Fish (2005, Chapter 5), and refer readers who are unfamiliar with reflection to this chapter and to the work of Donald Schön.

The following are the key points that we would make about reflection:

- It is a rigorous and disciplined form of enquiry into a piece of practice.
- The speaker/writer has to have been personally involved in that piece of practice.
- The talking and writing focuses on the writer's own role in the event.
- Being autobiographical, this talking and writing:
  - uses the first-person singular
  - is about concrete situations
  - seeks to understand the action/event which has been personally experienced
  - is 'in the moment' and enables the hearer/reader to feel that they were there
  - attends in detail to the context of the action/event being reflected on
  - seeks to study an event/action more deeply and to unpack the thinking and knowing beneath its surface
  - describes wholes rather than parts
  - is narrative in style and form
  - shows evidence of learning (deepening understanding)
  - sometimes uses rich and vivid descriptions based on, for example, comparisons (as in similes and metaphors)
  - demonstrates commitment to professional ideals and uses these as a touchstone to critique practice

- takes account of the views and perspectives of others involved in the action or event
- identifies factors contributing to the situation that may be historical, political, economic, social, ethical, autobiographical or psychological
- draws attention to what may previously have been taken for granted, rendering the familiar strange
- enriches experience by the acquisition of new perspectives
- seeks relationships to wider theory and general principles.

We are finding that many new doctors now coming into postgraduate medical education are familiar with and comfortable about reflection of this kind. Their teachers are currently less so, but once they have grasped the principles listed above, they will not find the process difficult, and many will find it remarkably rewarding.

Our view is that teacher and learner should engage in spoken reflection as often as possible, but that the reflective writing should unpack in far more detail than required on the form, the invisibles associated with each of the procedures assessed by DOPs and the cases assessed by C-bD. This would make in all 12 pieces of writing per year. We are confident that the very process of writing will enable learners to see more in the event than they realized before they began to write. That is, the learning is *in* the writing. The clinical supervisor will need to respond to at least some of these pieces (as many as seems appropriate and possible), by adding written comments that offer a response, and signing and dating them.

The reflective section of the portfolio, now apparently extant in all new medical curricula, is the proper place for the learner to collect – and the supervisor to read and comment on and sign – a summary of developing insights that have emerged in each attachment. The individual pieces should be filed elsewhere, but be made available if there is a challenge to the validity of the public summary. The fact that these reflections are on procedures and cases that learners have already spoken about with clinical supervisors or other assessors guarantees that the reflections are genuine and personal to the writer. The names and identities of patients and colleagues must of course be disguised on paper.

The importance of narrative in using the invisibles

As one of us (Fish 1998, p. 154) wrote several years ago:

> 'For the professional, story telling and hearing has some particularly important roles to play in helping us to understand our clients and in helping us to explore our own practice. These are stories that we tell and hear, but which, at the same time we are also part of. And we learn early in professional practice, if not in our early life, that there is always more than one version of a story. This, of course can be turned to positive use in trying to understand something through a story. And one of the things that we can learn to understand better is the art of story telling itself.'

We are not alone in emphasizing the importance of narrative in medicine. As Greenhalgh and Hurwitz (1998, p. 5), point out, 'not only do we live by narrative, but, often with our doctors and nurses as witnesses, we fall ill, get better, get worse, stay the same and finally die by narrative too.' They also point out (p. 7) that:

'● in the diagnostic encounter narratives are the form through which patients express their ill health, encourage empathy and promote understanding between clinician and patient, allow the construction of meaning, and offer analytical clues
● in the therapeutic process narratives encourage a holistic approach to management, are themselves intrinsically therapeutic or palliative, and may suggest ... additional therapeutic options
● in the education of patients and professionals narratives are often memorable, are grounded in experience, and enforce reflection
● in research, narratives set a patient-centred agenda, challenge received wisdom, generate new hypotheses.'

There is often much to disentangle in stories, and this is their entertainment value, provided the narrators have persuaded the audience early on to care about or identify with some aspects of the characters and the plot. Some of the key elements of narrative are that it has form and that the form should be appropriate to, and will shape and control how the audience interprets, the content. Stories have tellers and audience (with different viewpoints), a range of characters involved in the action (with varying interpretations of it) and sometimes a fictional observer or observers (who see the story from different perspectives).

Stories have context and plot, as well as time sequences, both as unfolding events (the sequence of events that happened in the story) and as events unfolded (the sequence in which we are told the story). This is a way of shaping whether the story is about what happened or about why it happened. There are some elements of a story that are relevant and some that are irrelevant to the main events. Stories are about people, with whom the audience quickly develops a relationship. They engage the audience and invite a response.

For doctors, who have to make sense of individual accounts of patients or of colleagues, in a world of complexity, paradox and ambiguity, above and beyond all else, stories:

● exist in the particular (they are about individuals)
● highlight the importance of moral enquiry (they show the importance of seeking in the given case what the most opportune action might be)
● promote the pursuit of practical reasoning – 'the ability to determine the best action to take in particular circumstances that cannot be distilled into universally applicable solutions' (Montgomery, 2006, p. 43).

Narrative is the vehicle for case-based discussion, and structures accounts of the engagement in medical techniques and procedures. These stories are told in order to fill in the assessment forms, but the record made does no justice to the level of insight and understanding brought to the case or the procedure by the learning doctor. That is why we think that a record of reflections on the invisibles is so important. Readers who wish to pursue the study of narrative in more detail are referred to Abbott (2002), Fish (1998, Chapters 6 and 7), Greenhalgh and Hurwitz (1998b) and Montgomery (2006).

But how will learners remember all these elements in the heat of practice and how will this help them to understand their practice better? We have twinned these invisibles with an image that will act as a prompt to help learners to remember them. The following introduces these.

THE HEURISTICS: A DEFINITION AND HOW THEY RELATE TO THE INVISIBLES

Basically, a heuristic is a memorable image that prompts us to explore and develop our understanding. It differs from a *framework* in that a framework holds a learner within the ideas it offers, asks that learner to work within those ideas, and is often relatively simplistic and one-dimensional in its focus. By contrast, a heuristic, being a picture, offers an open starting point or prompt for beginning to explore and develop understanding. That is, it provides an impetus for exploration that does not constrain how the learner then moves forward.

Our heuristics seek to provide three things:

- a memorable picture that will come to mind even during practice and that prompts exploration of understanding
- some language in which to unpack and explore the ideas that lurk beneath the implicit and tacit in practice
- an open approach to thinking through what is going on in one's mind, heart, body and soul as one engages in practice.

A heuristic prompts a complex, rich and honest exploration, and thus development, of understanding. We are particularly concerned to use these to help doctors develop and hone their professional judgements by understanding both how they come to those judgements and what drives them.

We have developed what we call a suite of heuristics, each of which is related to each of the invisibles. The aim of these is to help postgraduate medical practitioners (both learners and their teachers) to think out in detail and to open out to critique what underlies how they decide on treatment and talk with the patient about it. This involves making explicit what drives or affects the decisions they make. We believe that images are likely to provide a good and memorable heuristic device for this purpose.

Each chapter in this book, then, from 4 to 10, focuses on one of the seven invisibles and offers a heuristic to prompt the learner to remember it and a range of resources to enable learners to explore their own practice more deeply. Each chapter is self-standing. They can be used in any order. The principle involved is that the topic chosen for exploration has both arisen from the learner's own practice and makes sense (or is made to make sense) as part of a sequence of learning, rather than being an isolated topic with no relevance to the learner's current needs and interests or the teacher's educational responsibilities.

Developing the Wise Doctor

Table 2.1 gives an overview of the invisibles and their accompanying heuristics.

The prompt (or heuristic) is designed to provide a picture that will trigger in the learner's memory the particular invisible element it is associated with. Further, the representative letters for each heuristic make up a mnemonic that may act as an additional prompt: The mnemonic is a reminder that:

PERCHES on the doctor's shoulder at the **BEDSIDE** and **BEYOND**.

Table 2.1 An overview of the invisibles and their accompanying heuristics

The invisible element of practice and the chapter that explores it	The prompt and the letter(s) associated with it
The context, including the doctor's personal qualities as they affect the practice context CHAPTER 4	A drawing in imitation of a Monet painting **(P)**
The doctor's professional values CHAPTER 5	An acronym to remind us of the extended and restricted professional **(ER)**
The forms of knowledge the doctor draws upon CHAPTER 6	A set of cards containing the forms of knowledge **(C)**
The clinical thinking the doctor engages in CHAPTER 7	A helicoid whose complex pathways illustrate those of clinical thinking **(HE)**
The professional judgements the doctor makes CHAPTER 8	A picture of a see-saw representing the problems of balancing conflicting priorities **(S)**
The therapeutic relationship the doctor establishes with the patient CHAPTER 9	A Picasso painting depicting the doctor at the patient's bedside **(BEDSIDE)**
The doctor's ability to use reflection to deepen and extend understanding of all the social and clinical aspects of practice CHAPTER 10	A photograph of a complex clinical event reminding the doctor to look beyond that which has become familiar **(BEYOND)**

RELATING THE INVISIBLES TO THE 'TOOLS OF THE TRADE'

Figure 2.1 indicates where we see the key uses of 'Tools of the Trade' and where we would argue the invisibles should begin to take precedence. It should be noted that C-bD and DOPS began life at undergraduate level and that we are suggesting the introduction of the invisibles at the beginning of the foundation programme and their substitution for 'Tools of the Trade' by the end of the early years of specialty training.

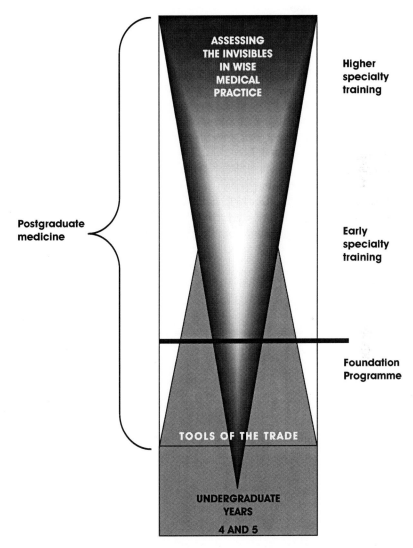

Figure 2.1   The roles of 'Tools of the Trade' and the invisibles in postgraduate medical education.

It should be noted that we provide in the Appendix a further table that offers a final overview of the relationship between the 'Tools of the Trade' and the resources offered in this book. It demonstrates how the resources provided for each invisible element contribute to the assessment of wise practice, and how this compares with what 'Tools of the Trade' can achieve. We have placed it in an appendix in order to separate it from any individual chapter because we believe that readers may wish to refer to it from time to time as they use the book.

FURTHER READING

Abbott, H Porter (2002) *The Cambridge Introduction to Narrative*. Cambridge: Cambridge University Press.

de Cossart L, Fish D (2005) *Cultivating a Thinking Surgeon: New Perspectives on Clinical Teaching, Learning and Assessment*. Shrewsbury: tfm Publications: Chapter 5.

Fish D (1998) *Appreciating Practice in the Caring Professions: Refocusing Professional Development and Practitioner Research*. Oxford: Butterworth Heinemann: Chapters 6 and 7.

Greenhalgh T, Hurwitz B, eds (1998) *Narrative Based Medicine*. London: BMJ Books: Chapters 17 and 18.

Montgomery K (2006) *How Doctors Think*: *Clinical Judgement and the Practice of Medicine*. Oxford: Oxford University Press: Chapter 3.

Schön D (1987a) *Educating the Reflective Practitioner*. New York: Jossey Bass: Chapters 1 and 2.

3

Principles for using learning resources: Teaching strategies, and the importance of talking and writing

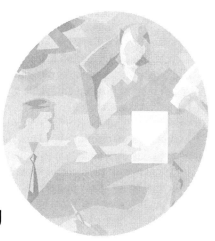

INTRODUCTION

The clinical setting has always been a rich resource for teaching postgraduate doctors. But much of that teaching has been 'on the hoof', opportunistic and lacking sequence, leaving trainees to make the best sense they can of the individual gems they pick up at random, and struggling to find a way of interrelating them. This has been termed 'the magpie approach to learning' (Brigley *et al.*, 2004), and has been (perhaps unthinkingly) accepted as 'the traditional way to do it'. This is not surprising, given the huge pressures on doctors' time, very little of which was seen as directly educational. We believe that this view has, until now, closed medical educators' eyes to the need for a more principled approach to the important activity of teaching junior doctors in the clinical setting. Further, since the new curricula now emerging have recast the clinical setting as the central arena for postgraduate education, a new look at teaching strategies has become inevitable.

Until now, clinical supervisors may be forgiven for not embarking on this apparently more demanding version of education. They have been given no help with the different principles upon which it is based, no demonstration of the educational strategies available to support it, and no resources designed specifically to promote the new approach to learning that it expects. This book seeks to enable learners to work in a more sequenced way on their understanding of the elements that we argue are at the core of medicine, and teachers to develop a more coherent set of principles and strategies for facilitating this in the clinical setting.

This approach demands of the teacher some pre-preparation and planning. And it demands of the learner that they take much more responsibility for their learning. But this is not the additional heavy burden that some seem to think. In fact, once the teacher understands the principles and strategies (and given that this book provides them with some rich resources for use by the learner), the pressure on teaching time will be reduced and the evidence now required for portfolios will develop naturally. Further, these approaches to education are familiar to many of the younger doctors entering service, so that there will, in most cases, be little need to 'sell' or explain the processes to them.

Teaching is fun, and so is learning – but only if the learner is actively involved, and only if the teaching is designed with a view to extending the learner's understanding by setting up enjoyable challenges that are calculated to demonstrate to teacher and learner alike the progress being made. This transfers considerable responsibility to the learner's shoulders, and requires them do some of the work as preparation or follow-up. This, inevitably, involves the learner in more writing and reading as preparation. But the learner who prepares more thoroughly for the interaction with the clinical supervisor can both offer more to it, and gain more from it. The great advantage of this is that coincidentally it builds sound evidence that can be made visible to teachers, learners and others who assess the learner's progress.

In this chapter, therefore, we seek to show what we mean by 'thinking like a teacher', rather than like a clinician who aims to present 'gems' to the learner. We explain the principles that underpin the new approaches to teaching in the clinical setting, we set out some strategies that teachers can employ to help learners make use of the resources offered in this book, and we explore some perspectives on the role of talking and writing in learning, and in particular how they might be employed by trainee and clinical supervisor. Firstly, however, we offer our grounds for arguing that doctors who have taught for years nonetheless need to critique and refine their ideas about teaching and learning in the light of what we provide here.

TEACHING IN THE CLINICAL SETTING: ASSUMPTION AND REALITY

Medical practitioners expect to update, refine or replace their medical knowledge on a regular basis. They do not accept that because X cured Y successfully in the 1900s there is no need to seek and use better methods now. They do of course ask for the evidence to back the claim 'better'. Education is no different, except that the evidence there is not of a quantitative but of a qualitative nature. Evidence about teaching and learning is rarely found in randomized controlled trials. It is best revealed in the detailed and rich texture of records accrued about individuals' learning and development. The following offers evidence of this kind for our claim that teachers in postgraduate medicine need to review and develop their ideas about teaching and the methods they use.

Over the last five years, one of us has worked in two Deaneries, with over 40 consultants (clinical supervisors) who believed that they were already quite good at teaching in the clinical setting. They came from every main specialty in medicine. One exercise they engaged in looked at the texture of the language in their conversations with learners. In most cases (though not all, because some were part of a small research project that had a continuity of its own), the conversations were examples of opportunistic teaching close to or in the clinical setting. These mostly followed up and reflected upon activities relating directly to patient care. As a consequence of this inevitably pragmatic response to learners' immediate needs, the logical sequencing, continuity, progression and development of educational provision (as enshrined in a curriculum) was largely missing. All the supervisors came to recognize this. (How to provide for this is illustrated in principle in the next section of this chapter and in detail in the scenarios that top and tail Chapters 4–10.)

Every one of the consultants had their assumptions about the quality of their teaching challenged, when brought face to face with the concrete evidence that they themselves had generated. This evidence was generated as follows.

Firstly, they were asked to express their educational intentions and beliefs about what they offer within the supervisory educational conversations they have with trainees in or near the clinical setting. Here is a typical example of the rather general writing that was done at this stage:

Consultant X

My educational intentions and my expectations were that I would be the main educational resource and a model. I would provide information at the right level for the trainee. And I would tell the trainee about other sources of information. I would look at their needs and respond to them. I hope I would also be brave enough to admit anything I do not know.

I expect my trainee to learn from the session; be prepared to engage in discussion with me; and to identify areas that need more attention.

Even at this point, it became clear to an experienced teacher's eye that consultants were not naturally 'thinking like teachers', who would have offered clear aims about how the learner would benefit from the session and how it would relate to previous and later ones. Rather, the consultants relied on their confidence as experienced clinicians who were able on the spot to talk about any clinical presentation, but without linking it into a sequence of learning. Thus, they talked in general terms, seeing teaching as offering their experience and the learner as automatically benefiting from it. They did not see teaching from the perspective of the learner. They did not think about facilitating learning.

Next, they captured (taped or videoed) a one-to-one professional conversation that was chosen because they believed it to be educational for the learner, it was about clinical practice and it took place within the clinical environment. Before replaying the tapes/DVDs, they jotted down what they thought had been achieved in their session. In every case, they have been very surprised, on first hearing or seeing the recording, at the difference between what they thought they had achieved and what actually happened. Consultant A's response was typical:

> **Consultant A**
> Immediately after the session, my first sensation was of relief. I had overestimated the obstacles in recording the session. I was surprised how easy it was to make a recording and how little note we took of the recorder once we began talking.
>
> I *thought* the session went well. We covered what I set out to do. I thought we consolidated his learning by using a clinical case in detail. But when I heard it back, I wasn't so pleased. I seemed to be doing all the work. And I have no idea what he took away with him. I even did the summary at the end, though I didn't mean to!

After this, consultants were encouraged to select (or in some cases we selected for them) a section of the tape/DVD and invited them to transcribe it (see Chapter 10 for more details of this process), and analyze the interaction from both an educational point of view and from the learner's point of view. This involved asking the following of the transcript, and seeking evidence (explicit or tacit) to support their answers:

- What was my implicit agenda here, and did I share my explicit educational intentions with the learner?
- What was the learner's agenda here, and did I hear or sense it and respond to it?
- What values and educational principles actually lie beneath this extract from my teaching, and how do these compare with my intentions for and assumptions about this conversation and about professional conversations generally?
- What does the learner do and what does the learner gain from this conversation, and how does this match what I assumed the learner would be doing and gaining?
- How did the learner actually see the conversation? (Ask them.)

All consultants were surprised – and many were fairly shocked – at what this revealed. The following offers some typical examples of what they wrote, slightly adapted for the sake of anonymity:

> **Consultant A (as above)**
> And the transcript was worse! The learner was clearly worried about something else altogether. At the start of our conversation, he makes several attempts to ask me about a procedure he had just carried out and that he was obviously uneasy about. But I just kept telling him it was OK, and rushed on to my main subject ...

> **Consultant B**
> ... All this shows that I overdirected the conversation and I was struggling to get the learner to understand *my* key points and why they

were important to me. But it also shows that though I have *listened* to the words and responses of the learner, I seem not to have *heard or understood* what the learner was saying or trying to say. Ironically, then, I was assuming that the learner (as he listened to me) was better than I at hearing the meaning behind words ...

Consultant C

I expected this to be a reasonably constructive conversation, and that we had explored the topic usefully. I wanted to encourage him to talk, but I now see that it would seem to him that I just kept shutting down on what he offered.

Consultant D

The more I read it, the more uncomfortable I got. The few bits where I did encourage and sustain him were minimal compared with what seems to me now to be repetitive and even insensitive or poorly worded questions that seemed to be about him guessing what I was thinking.

Consultant E

I like to think I will do this better another time, by getting her to clarify and summarize the issues and exploring her assumptions much further. I need to get learners to clarify, query, challenge, reshape their thinking ... or even to ask me for clarification.

Consultant F

... I see from this transcript new opportunities for learning/teaching that were not recognized at the time:

- things that could have been expanded on
- clues from the learner that I simply did not pick up
- seeking the answer already in my head and therefore not listening to the learner's reply
- not working with the answer supplied by the learner.

Consultant G

... This learner has a number of erroneous beliefs about the treatment for this kind of disease. I need to find a way of getting her to express and explore these so that her understanding is really extended. I did not do that on this occasion.

Consultant H

An unexpected finding for me was that the learner's explanation [of this process and why the patient was ill] was a complete misunderstanding of the whole thing – but I greeted it as if the overall explanation was correct, just the detail was wrong. ... I was very surprised at my lack of consistency in listening ... it was as if once the learner got the point, I relaxed and agreed with a number of incorrect assertions.

I also find it hard to maintain my own line of logic and at the same time to give the learner space and time to sort out his thinking and express it. It is a difficult balance to find ...

Many of the consultants who engaged with this were then offered the following models of teaching, which clarified for them the differences between these 'traditional' views of presentational teaching and other ways of working.

THREE DIFFERENT MODELS OF TEACHING – AND THE PRINCIPLES THAT UNDERPIN THEM

There are at least three ways of thinking about education (Table 3.1). Each of these differs sharply in terms of: their educational values; their assumptions about the role of the teacher, the learner and assessment; the kinds of resources needed; and the uses made of these resources by teacher and/or learner. If postgraduate medical education is to be successful in the future, clinical supervisors will need to know about and understand the implications of these differences

The traditional approach: the product or transmission model of education

The traditional way of teaching in postgraduate medicine both in the classroom and in the clinical setting is represented in the first column of Table 3.1. This assumes that the teacher should be an active transmitter of medical knowledge (which is seen as a product created by tradition and handed on by the teacher) and that the learner's central role is to absorb this 'product' and be able to regurgitate it on demand – both in exams and for the benefit of decision-making in clinical practice.

This model, as Fish and Coles (2005, p. 68) point out, values the teacher as an expert and knowledge as a fixed package. Here, everything (the roles of teacher and learner, the motivation, the resources and the key headings for planning) are about 'the learner gaining something visible that someone else has deemed important for them to have or know'. In this model, it is assumed that the teacher should be able to describe beforehand exactly what knowledge the learner will gain. The role of assessment is then to check at the end of the process that the learner has indeed acquired this. Here, knowledge is a product to be transferred from teacher to learner, which is why this is referred to as the product model. The main resource and source of information is the teacher, and learners are expected to learn by listening. This will be familiar to consultants, who often experience young doctors' expectations that a teaching session is about 'being told'. The product system is driven by exams, and doctors may wish to consider the effect that exams have on the whole of postgraduate medical education.

The product model will be a very familiar way of thinking about teaching for all readers. It is, after all, how most consultants were taught in school and university – though it is not the way more recent medical graduates learn. But we should remember that it was designed for use in classrooms, where the sole intention was to pass on subject knowledge, and where the ultimate assessment process was usually by national examinations. Further, the only agenda that mattered was the teacher's, and the main activities were teacher talking and learners both listening and making extensive notes for themselves, ready to write at greater length for assessment purposes. Whilst this model might offer a basis for postgraduate lectures (and will always be one of the ways of offering the learner new knowledge), clearly it does not provide all that is necessary for the clinical supervisor who is teaching in the practice setting. Here, there is no time for extensive lectures by the teacher. Here what is taught involves practical processes, complex thinking, and the appropriate selection and use of theoretical knowledge. This draws the learner into active participation. Thus, in the practice setting, a different model is required.

The approach to teaching required by new postgraduate medical curricula (the process model)

In the new approach to education now being introduced in postgraduate medicine, the teaching and assessment that take place in the clinical setting have been made the central thrust. Now, teaching has to be more sequenced than opportunistic, and practical assessments must be more carefully recorded. This requires an approach to education that is based on the process model of teaching.

Here, the processes referred to are those of the learner. This model values a learner who is active and more responsible for his or her own learning, whose own agenda is of interest to the teacher, and who engages more interactively with the teacher. These are detailed in the second column of Table 3.1. The aim is to help the learner to seek knowledge and, in addition, to gain understanding and make it appropriate to their own context by working actively with it. Thus the roles of both teacher and learner are more collaborative, though the teacher is still an agent for knowledge that comes from 'above'. This means that while a proper postgraduate 'criticality' is built into this model – in that practice is critiqued in the light of theory – the theory is often left unchallenged and taken as 'given'. The learning here is active, and assessment takes place during and as part of the learning, and its role is to help both teacher and learner to see current achievements and thus to design and re-design the processes of teaching and learning in the light of the learner's progress.

In this model, the quality of the learning becomes apparent by charting the learner's increasing insight and understanding (and consequent conduct) over a period of time. Resources are the central driving force in this model. They should offer learners ways of exploring new ideas, meeting new language, and working

Table 3.1 Three models of teaching, learning and assessment (based upon the ideas of Stenhouse, 1975)[a]

Education as a product	Education as a process	Education as research
Intention: Teacher transmits knowledge	*Intention:* Teacher promotes knowledge	*Intention:* Learners explore understanding
Locus of knowledge: Resides in teacher	*Locus of knowledge:* Resides in teachers and learners	*Locus of knowledge:* Resides in learner group
Student activities: Passive learners (covers material fast)	*Student activities:* Active learners (active learning takes longer)	*Student activities:* Aware of selves as active learners and negotiators (this takes even longer)
Motivation via: Teacher	*Motivation via:* Own active learning	*Motivation via:* Group learning/active learning
Sees learner as: Receiver of knowledge	*Sees learner as:* Active seeker of knowledge	*Sees learner as:* Discoverer/reconstructor of own knowledge
Sees teacher as: Teller/instructor	*Sees teacher as:* Seeker/catalyst	*Sees teacher as:* Facilitator/neutral chair
Teaching activities: Lecturing	*Teaching activities:* Facilitates learning Sets up problems Probably knows answers	*Teaching activities:* Teacher is leader within group but learns alongside them

Sees assessment as: End-of-course tests, Summative, Teacher assessment	*Sees assessment as:* Part of teaching, Part of learning, Formative – and summative	*Sees assessment as:* Self-assessment, Group assessment, Aiding understanding
Plans by means of: Aims, Objectives, Detailed method for whole session, Summative assessment	*Plans by means of:* Aims, Intentions, Principles of procedure, List of content, Assessment as part of this process	*Plans by means of:* Aims, Intentions, A negotiated agenda, Counselling-type methods, Assessment within this process
Use of resources: Chosen by teacher and brought into the learner's context from outside by the teacher, and thus may not relate to learner's context	*Use of resources:* Learner-centred, and thus inevitably arising from the learner's context and relevant to it	*Use of resources:* Learner organized, and thus chosen from the learners' context
View of professional: Teacher is a performer whose performance is significant in the quality of learners' education	*View of professional:* Teacher/facilitator sets up learning for learners and makes less input in the sessions	*View of professional:* Facilitator/teacher learns alongside learners, but this can only be on a highly disciplined basis

[a]Adapted from Fish and Coles (2005, pp. 69–70).

at their own pace and level, to increase their understanding. Sessions with the teacher will then involve discussions at a higher level where the learner's new thinking and insights are consolidated, refined, challenged and related to the learner's current practice (see Fish and Coles, 2005, pp. 68–70).

The process model demands a shift in the burden of work from teacher to learner, because the main resources offered by the teacher are used by the learner to prepare for or follow up the time spent with the teacher. This means that the learner works without the teacher (at his/her own pace and in the way preferred) and *then* meets the teacher, who now becomes a means of checking out the understanding and awareness of the implications of the resources offered. Further, the main speaker for much of this meeting is the learner, while the teacher becomes substantially the listener and by this means is more sure of what the learner is understanding and how he/she is progressing.

In the examples from consultants' own investigations of their teaching given above, there are clear signs of them moving gradually from the product model of teaching to the process model. This can be found in their awareness of their predominating voice, in their recognition that learners should be doing more, and in their frustration at not knowing what these learners think and understand.

Beyond this, however, there is a third model that we predict will ultimately influence some of the learning in the clinical setting, and that we take up in more detail in Chapter 10. This is known as the research model.

The approach to teaching for future use in postgraduate medicine: the research model

The research model of learning and teaching is in a sense an extension of the process model, and will probably grow out of it naturally as new ways of teaching in postgraduate medicine continue to develop. It can be seen in the third column of Table 3.1. This model heightens and values particularly the *investigative* aspects that we have described above in the process model, and a wider criticality. As Fish and Coles (2005) say, this model 'sees the aim as enabling learners to explore understanding and to become emancipated from knowledge "handed down" to them'. It follows that in this model the resources are used for extending understanding, inviting new theories, and critiquing not only practice in the light of theory but also theory in the light of practice. Here the relevant resources are increasingly found by the learner, not given by the teacher – see the third column of Table 3.1. Chapter 10 offers some detailed examples of how this might work. Because this model emphasizes the need for discovery, critique and investigation by the learner, it is more challenging for the teacher who cedes power to the learner. But it is more enjoyable, because both partners become learners together in uncharted waters.

The need for resources and teaching strategies

We would argue that teachers and learners working in postgraduate medicine for the 21st century will need, as a minimum, to adopt the principles of the process model and to work towards the research model. The educational principles involved in both these models make *high-quality learning resources* the key to success. This also demands that teachers develop strategies for directing learners in how to use these most beneficially. We are anxious to point out, however, that what we are commending here is not in any way a form of distance learning. It still places regular face-to-face interaction with the teacher at the centre of the learning process. It is best achieved in a 'safe clinical practicum' (de Cossart and Fish, 2005, p. 60).

The final section of this chapter provides an example of the kind of sequence of stages that we believe is needed to 'bring to life' this resource-based learning. It also highlights the role of talking and writing in this process.

TEACHING STRATEGIES AND LEARNING RESOURCES: TURNING TEACHING INTO LEARNING IN THE CLINICAL SETTING

In turning teaching into learning, so that the learner becomes the more active of the parties, talking will be the main vehicle for exploration when the teacher is present, and writing and reading will be the activities in which the learner needs to engage, in preparation for and follow-up to the discussion with the consultant. This will make for a very different form of conversation with the consultant, and will involve the learner in various kinds of writing, using either bullet points or a more extended form. This writing (which in most cases will be brief) will primarily be for the learner, will aid both teacher and learner to see what has been made of the resources, ideas and language offered, and will form the basis of evidence for the learner's portfolio.

Since much of the skill here is in designing and setting up the work of the learner, we look first in detail at that. We then consider in some detail the processes of talking and writing, asking what range of strategies the teacher can use to promote them.

Setting up the task to get the most out of the resources available

Resource-based learning, in our experience, is best served by a sequence of activities, which involve the clinical supervisor and a single learner or a small group of two or three learners. Typically, these stages would be:

1. The spotting of an appropriate learning opportunity
2. A brief meeting to agree how learner(s) should prepare for a discussion with their clinical supervisor
3. Private preparation by the learner(s)
4. The professional conversation between teacher and learner(s) to ensure the development of learners' ideas
5. A written follow-up on this topic by learner(s) on their own

6. A review by teacher and learner of the record of what has been learnt from this event.

The learner here will be the postgraduate doctor in training, who is usually still called the 'trainee', but whom we prefer to call 'the learner' since we are concerned with education rather than training. The teacher will be the clinical supervisor or any other doctor or other senior professional who teaches the learner in the clinical setting. In addition, from time to time, the educational supervisor (as distinct from the clinical supervisor) may contribute a seventh stage to the process by reviewing the learner's development. This will involve exploring with the learner a summary of key learning points across a given period, for which the learner's portfolio provides more detailed evidence.

The finer details of this are now provided below.

Stage 1: Spotting the learning opportunity

Either the teacher or the learner (but initially the teacher) needs to be seeking at all times while working in the clinical setting, a clinical event *that teacher and learner have shared* and that can be used as a trigger to enable both of them to explore something that fits the learner's current sequencing (level and stage) of learning, as specified in, or appropriate to, their learning agreement. This means that it should be something that is both rich enough to raise important issues or principles of clinical care and related enough to other recently studied topics, so as to render it more broadly important than if it were merely an isolated 'gem' of interest. In other words, the event spotted will be particularly significant and will repay considerable study, having both the potential to be explored in depth (perhaps to support immediate patient care) and also offering important ideas and issues worth consideration at the level of principle. Spotting these opportunities is something of a skill. And like all skills, it is best developed in practice and in the light of reflections upon that practice with the intent of refining it.

We would suggest that most learning opportunities will arise within clinical cases where the learner has been closely involved and is able to see the unrolling of the clinical event in detail. Here, the trigger is the element of the case that is significant for the learner's agenda. The first stage in such a teaching sequence might then be to fill in a case-based discussion form. The teacher's role here is to ensure that the case selected is appropriate.

Stage 2: Agreeing how learner(s) should prepare for a discussion with their clinical supervisor

This stage is crucial in providing the firm foundation for the success of the rest of the teaching stages. It requires a brief meeting between teacher and learner(s), to set up each learner's preparation and clarify the tasks so that the rest of the teaching and learning time is spent profitably. This could take place as soon as the case-based discussion form has been filled in. It involves the following:

1. Inviting the learner(s) to engage in resource-based learning – not as a coercion, but as offering the promise of learning together and motivating the learner to prepare for this

2. Recognizing and articulating together how the topic, in terms of content and activity, fits the learner's learning needs. This means shaping the educational goals so that they are relevant and achievable and everyone is working in the same direction, but without shutting out new directions that may arise as the work continues. This should ensure that the learner is clear how this work follows on from previous work, relates to present clinical experience and will lead on to future development

3. Setting up the preparatory work that the learner will engage in, so that there is no misunderstanding about the task (which should involve critique of theory and of practice), and no puzzlement about the resources offered to support it and how they should be used. This may mean offering an example of how to set out the writing required

4. Fixing (and privileging) a date and time for the face-to-face discussion.

By these simple means, the learner is provided with a sense of continuity (so often missing in learning in the clinical setting), and with a strong sense that the work he/she will do will be acknowledged and valued. A final act of support might be to indicate where learners can find the teacher at an interim time should they still be doubtful about what to do.

Long as this description of the process is, it takes relatively little 'real time', being completed in most cases within 15 or so minutes. But this will only be the case if the resources are ready to hand and the teacher has done a little thinking ahead about the potential of the event, the overall aim(s) of the teaching sequence, the focus of the professional conversation (Stage 4) and the design of the tasks to make the most of the learning opportunity.

Stage 3: Private preparation by the learner(s)

The learner's preparation may be solo or with peers, but is without a teacher. In this stage, learners need to use the learning resources (which might include their peers) to the full. This requires a willingness to confront and explore new ideas and even new language, but at least this can be done at the learner's own pace. The intention is to enable each learner to make their own meaning out of the materials and to think about how these relate to their current clinical practice. They then need to find and prepare a means of conveying to others the new under-standings and insights into their own practice that they have gained.

Stage 4: The meeting for a professional conversation to ensure the development of learners' ideas

The meeting with the clinical supervisor is the opportunity to share and check out the new ideas gained. These need to be challenged and extended by the clinical supervisor – and, where relevant, by peers who are part of the teaching group.

Developing the Wise Doctor

The teacher's opening words here are crucial in setting a safe environment in which learners can reveal and explore frankly the results of their work. The clinical supervisor should think carefully about how to begin, and, if there is more than one learner, who to begin with. It is also important not to damage this nurturing environment by insensitive responses to the learner's offerings.

Here the more traditional roles are reversed, the teacher becoming more of a listener, and learners talking more. But what is significant is that they can now offer in discussion higher levels of understanding than they would have done without the preparation, and since the level of discussion is raised, the time spent with the consultant can be used more profitably. This means that seriously new meanings, insights and understandings can be created 'in the air between learners and the teacher', and that both parties are working creatively, enjoyably and for mutual gain. Indeed, the teaching and learning possibilities that can arise from the educational task that has been set are bounded only by the scope of the educational imagination of the teacher and learner, who, even as they proceed on a chosen task, may find themselves creating new ideas both about the task and about where it can take them. It is this that makes education an adventure. It is – very properly – less predictable, and inevitably more rewarding than 'training' (which, un-inspiringly for the bright doctor, sets ahead of the game what it is that will be learnt and achieved).

Stage 5: A written follow-up on this topic by learner(s) on their own

The follow-up session is the opportunity for the learner to capture, consolidate and develop further in writing the new understandings that have been reached and the new insights that have been gained, and to speculate about how they will use these in future practice. Of course, this is not as simple as 'putting new learning straight into next practice', because the context of each clinical event renders it specific and un-generalizable, and because putting into practice something one has learnt is not as easy or as simple as it sounds. New experience and insight nonetheless underpin wise practice, because these are the resources that doctors feed into their new thinking about each new patient.

Stage 6: A review by teacher and learner of the record of what has been learnt from this event

The writing produced by the learner in follow-up should contain a dated summary, designed to be included in the portfolio. This summary should indicate the insights gained and developments achieved as a result of this teaching sequence. The clinical supervisor (or whoever has taught this sequence) should respond very briefly to this summary, in writing (dated and initialled) at the end of the learner's piece.

The teacher's comments should consist of no more than two or three sentences of 'appreciation' of the learner's achievements. It should be critical and if necessary corrective, but it should also 'recognize' as important any significant points made by the learner, and provide an indication of the teacher's overall impression of the writing. (The term 'appreciation' here echoes what happens in a walk through an art gallery, where certain pictures draw the attention, and significant elements of these are recognized and pointed out before an overall response to the whole picture is offered.)

The learner's summary and the supervisor's 'appreciation' of it will then be available for the review of the portfolio by the educational supervisor from time to time, and in particular, at the Record of In-Training Assessment (RITA) review.

The importance of 'differentiation'

Where more than one learner is going to be present in the discussion with the consultant, such learners are likely to be at very different career stages. Thus, their experience needs to be carefully taken into account so that, while all are contributing to a group focus, and will teach and learn from each other, the tasks they will prepare privately need to be properly *differentiated* across learners in relation to their different career stages and individual abilities.

'Differentiation' is a teaching term indicating that, within a group of learners who are working together but who are at very different levels of experience or ability, the teacher has appropriately graded the difficulty of the tasks set, to take account of each individual's level, while also maintaining a group approach to the topic, and, where possible, using each learner as a resource for the others.

Talking and listening for learning: some issues and strategies

Once the learner has prepared for the discussion with the consultant, this face-to-face interaction is a vital component to enable understanding to be identified, critiqued and developed. Dialogue by e-mail, while better than nothing, is no real substitute for picking up the nuances of meaning and the spontaneous development of new understanding that is found in professional conversations, and so there should always be a significant proportion of personal meetings. The conversation that this allows should be more enjoyable for both parties than 'feedback sessions', because the groundwork has been done and time can be used more profitably.

As we have already seen, in resource-based learning, the learner not only does more of the work, but during the professional conversation will probably need to talk more than the teacher. Learners use talk to present and discuss the new ideas and insights they have gained from the private preparation stage described above. By this means they begin to make these ideas – and the language in which they are best expressed – their own. In addition, they learn to challenge their own previous thoughts and assumptions and also discover themselves creating new understanding *as they talk*. That is the importance of talk. In talking, knowledge can never be transmitted simply, from one person to another. It has to be constructed afresh by each individual on the basis of what they already know, what they hear, and by means of strategies for gaining clarification, seeking explanation and offering new thoughts. Teachers and learners will have developed these strategies during life's ordinary conversations. In a dialogue, which is a kind of improvisation, we modify and amplify our ideas and their expression in the light of feedback, so that *meaning is jointly construed.* Thus talk allows for the reconstruction of knowledge during the conversation.

However, where the participants in a conversation come from different cultural backgrounds, or where they differ considerably in level of experience and knowledge, the possibility of misunderstanding is ever present. Teacher and learner therefore need to take care that the meanings constructed between them do not become increasingly divergent. Teachers should remember that:

- for every learner, a slightly different interpretation is placed on teacher's words
- learners need the chance to formulate and check out the sense they make of new topics
- teachers need to know what sense learners are making of what they offer
- this is a means of valuing explicitly what the learner brings to the learning.

For these reasons, the teacher needs to:

- listen carefully to what the learner says
- try to understand it from the learner's viewpoint
- take the learner's meanings as the basis for what he/she says next
- use vocabulary and syntax (word order) that the learner understands.

Thus, conversation between teacher and learner will become *collaborative.* Further, since knowledge can only be constructed by individual learners, who need at best to be actively engaged in all the processes involved, it is clear that we need a model of education based on *partnership* between teachers and learners, in which the responsibility for selecting and organizing the tasks to be engaged in is shared. Thus, the curriculum becomes negotiated; teachers become experts in facilitating learning, in guiding learners in re-inventing knowledge and in enriching their meaning-making; and learners begin to take control of their learning and can engage in self-assessment.

That is why we are arguing that opportunities for teacher to listen to learner need to be structured into the normal teaching/working context. But all listening should be for a clear purpose. For this to happen, the scene should be set to encourage an honest, highly motivated and brave discussion from which the learner will gain much. The words used by the consultant at all stages should establish a desire for a shared and cooperative learning session and set an atmosphere in which the learner has no reluctance in opening up their difficulties, hesitations and anxieties.

Indeed, we would argue that the key strategies used to draw the learners to think and to share their new idea(s) aloud are: *silence* and *space*! This may seem counterintuitive (the teacher is usually presumed to be there to 'tell' learners how to get it right, and not to waste time in leaving silences). But it works. By not coming in first with an evaluative comment, but holding back and waiting to see what sense the others have made of this, the teacher allows the learner a chance to show what they can do, and the teacher can learn more about where the learner is.

Good listening by the teacher for educational purposes related to developing the learner's understanding is a key to good teaching. However, the expertise involved in careful listening is often seriously underestimated, and is far more complex than it appears. Firstly, it is difficult for a teacher to listen rather than talk. Secondly, listening is not the same as hearing (what one person says and the other person hears are often shockingly different, as we showed earlier). Thirdly, the ability to listen is part of a highly complex process related to the individual, the context, and the listener's knowledge and experience, motivation and degree of involvement. The good listener:

- reaches out to understand what the talker is saying and holds back his/her own ideas, keeping them separate from what is being said and being careful not to let them interfere with either what the learner is expressing or the way he/she is expressing it
- listens until the end (or the end of an appropriate point) and neither switches off after a few seconds because the beginning sounds OK nor works on possible answers/counter-arguments/comments during the course of listening to the preclusion of hearing the whole argument
- listens for an educational *purpose* that is different according to whether the interaction is a debate (to win the point), a personal reflection on practice (to offer a supportive and critical ear) or a deliberative exploration (to encourage the speaker's creativity)
- listens supportively, because listeners can hugely affect the confidence of speakers, can control them and can even refuse to recognize their contribution (this includes alertness to one's own and the learner's body language)
- is non-judgemental and shows unconditional regard for the speaker (this does *not* preclude subsequent correction, if necessary, and a friendly criticality!)
- responds to the speaker in open and honest ways and shows this intention to the speaker early on
- regards any conversation as involving turn-taking, where both (all) parties work together to push out the boundaries of their understanding.

Listening involves hearing, concentration, understanding, responding, memory and motivation. It also involves receptive skills (i.e. accuracy of listening) and reflective skills (i.e. analysis, interpretation, relation of new to old material, criticality and appreciation). It involves sensitivity to phonology (i.e. vocabulary, stress and intonation, hesitation, pause, silence and volume). The slightest change in stress and intonation can lead to quite different meanings. Even a slight difference in pronunciation can change the word 'late' to 'light'; differences of stress can change 'one-armed bandit' to 'one armed bandit'; differences in intonation provide the difference between a question, a statement, a hesitation, an uncertainty or an exclamation. Listening also involves sensitivity to register (style, tone and rhythm). Register enables us to recognize a number of different contexts (technical/non-technical, formal/informal, impersonal/personal, literal/figurative, evaluative/uncritical, rational/emotional and public/private).

Having already appreciated more fully where the learners are and what they have already achieved (or how little they understand about something they have been assumed to know), the teacher can focus on the development of new ideas. It is a matter of professional judgement for the teacher when to press home his/her own agenda and when to pursue the agenda of the learner. What is important is to be aware of both agendas, and where appropriate to insist (with due support) on the learner moving on from preferred safe ground. For example, some learners do not easily shed the notion that they are being tested, and will 'duck out' of the challenge being offered and back into traditional, even ritualistic, talk, designed to return to an individual patient or to prepare for the exams.

The underlying principles here are that the discussion should be cooperative and positive in tone, that it should seek to acknowledge the learner's achievements and take the thinking on, and that when a breakthrough in learning occurs, it is recognized overtly by the teacher. One useful strategy is that, wherever possible, it should be the learner who makes the main points, and the learner who summarizes at appropriate stages in the conversation.

Summarizing as an example

Conversation is not scripted. It is actually a form of improvisation (Schön, 1987a). Conversations are not about the presentation of cut and dried 'knowledge' by one party to another who listens silently and then regurgitates back a briefer version of it. The whole point of learning conversations is that understanding is newly created and meaning is elaborated between teacher and learner, *during them*. Summarizing learning conversations therefore means giving a concise account of the arguments, clarifications and elaborations that arose during the discussion, and giving tongue to the new insights that the conversation has stimulated. It is often used at the end of a conversation, but can also be used profitably at appropriate points as the conversation develops.

Summarizing by the learner in all sorts of situations is a very useful way for teachers to find out what the learner knows and (more importantly) understands. Postgraduate doctors are assumed to be good at summarizing, but their skill is more to do with summarizing scientific facts in respect of patient cases (often at handover points in care). This is a check of knowledge. By contrast, giving a résumé of key points in a developing and creative educational discussion is about the learner's understanding. This is much harder than summarizing a patient case. This is not about facts. What is being summarized in a learning conversation is often the first attempt by both teacher and learner to respond to new thinking, express new arguments, and formulate new ideas. Elements of interpretation in respect of the meaning of words are bound to creep in at all points and may need further clarification, or correction if inaccurate material is imported into the summary. This will offer both parties a useful opportunity for further extension of their thinking. Indeed, the teacher who listens to a learner's summary and also the learner (who should be 'self-monitoring' what they say as they say it) should watch out for this opportunity. Even at the summary stage, meaning is made *between people* in a conversation. Thus, it should be clear that summarizing is not a test of the learner, but part of the learning process, which the teacher supports and may take part in. However, it is fair to alert learners at the start of the discussion that their role will include leading the summarizing.

Thus, summarizing gives the learner a chance to check that he/she has understood, gives the teacher a chance to clarify any key points still not picked up and helps both teacher and learner to relate new ideas to ones already held, and to critique both the new and old.

When a good point has been made in summary, it may be worth writing down. Learners can then be sure to come away from a conversation with their grasp of both new information and new and complex ideas checked out. This in turn raises issues about how important it is for learners to write down key points, and about when and to what end this should be done.

Writing for learning in the clinical setting: some issues and strategies

Writing is not merely a way of recording learning that has been completed. Indeed, when used this way, it is a rather sterile activity, and exams are an example of this. Writing is also (much more interestingly) a way of *finding out* what you think and what you know. In that case, the learning occurs *in the writing* – it is not brought to the writing and merely recorded there. Rather, what matters is working over the writing in order to reshape it so as to make it express one's understanding as accurately as possible. In doing this, one clarifies and deepens that very understanding.

As we have already pointed out, writing is a useful way of preparing and following up a session with an expert. It is a means of crystallizing what has been learnt. Doctors already write for a wide variety of medical purposes. Writing for learning also needs to be part of their repertoire. Such writing can be in note form, or as bullet points, or in the shape of forms, charts, diagrams and posters, or presented as flowing prose. Writing reflectively is perhaps the most educationally useful form of 'flowing prose'. This should arise out of talking and thinking reflectively, and should be used from time to time to capture the complexities of cases or events that will repay particular scrutiny; de Cossart and Fish (2005, Chapter 5) provide further details of this. Table 3.2 is adapted from that chapter and illustrates the difference between talking and writing reflectively from a learner's perspective.

When using writing as part of resource-based learning, there should be a clear agreement between teacher and learner about the intentions, the content and the form of any writing task associated with using learning resources. The writing activities should be short but specific and achievable, and designed to engage and

Table 3.2 Talking and writing reflectively[a]

Talking reflectively	Writing reflectively
• Can be used to explore ideas and make them your own (can be dialogic)	• Often reveals more than you set out to say and teaches you what you think (can be dialogic)
• Can happen in the action	• Rarely occurs during action
• Is time-limited by events and ephemeral	• Is enduring and often leads to special satisfaction
• Is rough and ready	• Can be reshaped
• Is personal and seems 'subjective'	• Is personal but can seem more objective
• Is quick to produce and to hear	• Takes longer to write and to read
• Is unlikely to be perfectly ordered and clear	• Can be given shape and balance
• Cannot stop and look back over points made, and so cannot easily refine them	• Can review points at all stages, and so can refine them
• Is no good for exploring intricate ideas and complex arguments	• Can present arguments and connections more clearly because the written text allows for demonstrating the logic and for redrafting
• May not facilitate the comparison of many complex facts and figures	• Can make such comparisons easily and allows and records readjustment and refinement
• Means it is hard to hold enough in the head to keep all ideas coherent	• Hard copy allows the refinement of understanding
• Is face-to-face and very direct	• Enables you to express some things you could not easily say
• Means ideas are fragile; interruptions can cause loss of thought and progress can be blocked, especially for learners	• Is more robust; you can come back later, and add to it or refine or change it; ideas can be revisited.
• Means you can discover what you have to say as you go, but you have to be quick and can't unsay something once it has been said	• Allows more time to discover what you want to say and how best to say it
• Can be artistic in content and form – but only if rehearsed	• Can be artistic in content and form, and extends the power to find the right words, especially in redrafting
• Can be inhibited by the social context	• Enables you to adopt an unusual or private role

[a]Adapted from de Cossart and Fish (2005, Chapter 5).

motivate as well as provide the concrete resources for a well-informed later discussion. The writing task should be first and foremost centred on supporting teaching and learning, and only be used for assessment purposes afterwards, when it has become a record of progress.

Indeed, the good design of these activities is key to the success of the whole educational endeavour. Thus any task agreed will be carefully designed not as a formal assessment but to help learners to come to grips at their own speed with both the new ideas and language for considering them, and to get them ready for the planned developmental discussion, to capture evidence of where they have begun, as a baseline for this discussion, and to enable continuity of theme and thus of education. By this means, as these ideas grow and become more informed through later discussion, the learners and the teacher will be able to review the first learning task and recognize the progress demonstrated by greater success in subsequent tasks. In contrast to this, learners who engage only in discussion can be falsely persuaded at the end of it either that they have made no progress and have learnt nothing new (when in fact they have), or that their achievement is greater than it actually is.

Further, the learner's writing will provide, for a range of audiences (self, other portfolio readers, patients, general managers, colleagues, or risk managers), some irrefutable evidence of learning. By getting the learner to write down both what he/she already knows and thinks, and then asking for further exploration to be recorded and annotated in writing, the teacher is both establishing sound and lasting evidence (for them both to see and to consider) of the learner's starting points, learning needs and, ultimately, progress, and is ensuring that there are good concrete resources to aid learning through the later discussion.

Because of the design of this whole educational endeavour, learners are doing the work, becoming engaged in it, discovering for themselves (which is always more persuasive and memorable than 'being told' by someone else), 'teaching themselves', with some guidance, and learning how to begin to investigate practice that will ultimately enable them to take over their own personal development.

End-note

With these ideas in mind, the reader is now invited to consider the resources offered in the rest of this book, and also to think critically about the scenarios provided that exemplify how such resources may be used.

FURTHER READING

de Cossart L, Fish D (2005) *Cultivating a Thinking Surgeon: New Perspectives on Clinical Teaching, Learning and Assessment.* Shrewsbury: Tfm Publications: Chapter 4.
Passmore J (1998) *The Philosophy of Teaching.* London: Duckworth.

Part Two

Attending to the core of medicine: Key resources for exploring the invisibles

Introduction to Part Two

The second part of this book focuses on the invisibles of practice. Throughout Part Two, each chapter is designed to:

- provide all readers with a means of engaging in resource-based learning, which lies at the heart of the new curricula for the whole of postgraduate medical education from the Foundation Programme through to Higher Specialty training
- provide teachers with illustrative examples of teaching strategies and sound resources to offer the learner
- provide learners with ways of extending their understanding of the specific 'invisible' element and its relevance to clinical practice and to show how exploring this can lead to a refinement of that practice
- indicate that some of this thinking about practice can be done without the presence of the teacher (to the benefit of both teacher and learner)
- demonstrate that the teacher's input at certain points is vital for the success of this whole approach to learning.

Whilst the focus of the book is on resource-based learning, this does not ignore the importance of assessment and of keeping the learner's achievements and progress well documented. In fact, if the strategies suggested are followed and the resources are used thoroughly and rigorously, the assessment and documentation of progress will already have been taken care of. Then all that will be needed at the summative assessment point is a résumé of achievement across the required period.

Each chapter in Part Two follows broadly the same structure. They contain the following:

- an opening scenario to help readers to consider a real clinical event in the light of the resources offered in the chapter and to help teachers to see how to set up sequenced learning opportunities

- a set of questions that the chapter addresses explicitly or implicitly
- an introduction to the chapter topic and an explanation of why it is important for learning doctors
- a heuristic that provides a picture prompt to remind readers of the key issue
- a set of resources to enable teachers and learners to deepen and extend understanding about their work in the clinical setting
- a closing scenario and sometimes a commentary on it, both of which are designed to extend ideas for teaching and learning
- some further reading.

Teachers might be advised to work through the resources themselves before – or at least alongside – engaging the learner in them. 'Never offer learners a resource you haven't first tried out yourself' has always been considered a sound educational principle! Learners should recognize, amongst what is offered, those resources that they can use for themselves and those where they need their teacher's help.

The heuristics offered are designed as a prompt to help doctors as they work in the clinical setting to remember the key invisibles and to use them both to 'reflect in their practice' even while they are engaged in it, and to 'reflect on their practice' after the event. These terms were first coined by Schön and have become central to reflective learning throughout healthcare.

In the scenarios offered, teachers are either referred to as consultants or teachers, while learners are depicted as either Specialist Registrars (SpRs) or learning doctors. It should be noted that these are not meant to imply that the ideas in the book are only for SpRs and consultants. Individuals cope differently with different levels of demand, and resources can be scaled up or down in complexity (by adding some in or leaving some out). It is therefore impossible to make blanket statements about what should be used when. Thus we would argue that the ideas and resources in each chapter need to be deployed (initially at least by teachers), using professional judgement, to offer them at a range of levels.

We believe that the invisibles can certainly be revisited at different career stages as the clinical scene becomes more demanding, the dilemmas become commensurately more difficult and the learner needs to work at a higher and higher level (which is not about doing different things but about doing things differently).

Finally, we have one warning. The sign of a poor teacher is rushing to 'use up' all the resources at once. The resources are there to prompt deep thinking, not to encourage a fast journey through all the possible aspects of a topic in the quickest possible time. Those who try to 'cover the whole field' speedily will do so shallowly. Resources need to be used only when learners are at an appropriate stage to benefit fully from them because they relate to current needs and to the relevant curriculum stage. Then they need to be dwelt upon and savoured, revisited and reconsidered in an educational sequence of the kind illustrated in Chapter 3.

Readers are therefore cautioned not to use this as a textbook to be 'worked through' fast, but invited to treat it as a 'box of delights' to be dipped into at appropriate moments.

4

Being alert to the context of the patient case: Prompted by Heuristic 1

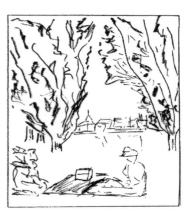

OPENING SCENARIO

You are invited to read this chapter with the following scenario in mind:

The trainee doctor's story: 'The morning after'
I was the Specialist Registrar (SpR) coming on duty at the city hospital. It was Sunday morning. I was told by the receptionist who was going off duty that it had been a busy night. She hoped that I would have a quiet day. I thanked her and put on my Accident and Emergency (A & E) suit. I poured myself a cup of coffee as I perused the list of patients on the board.

At 9 AM, I began the handover ward round with the SpR who had been on for the night, who looked tired and worn out, and the nurse in charge for the day. We started at the bed of a rather dishevelled looking young man. My SpR colleague presented him as a young man who was recovering from excess alcohol intake and who had injured his arm. His laceration had been sutured. He had no evidence of head injury, and the usual antibiotics and tetanus injections had been given. He had been abusive to the staff, but now seemed to have calmed down and was ready for discharge. A follow-up appointment at the dressings clinic was to be arranged. The SpR chided the young man about his excess alcohol intake. She also asked if there was anyone he wished us to contact. He replied firmly 'No'. The ward round moved on.

As we were approaching the next bed, a nurse came to say that the mother of the boy in the previous bed was in the visitor's room and was very upset. She wanted to speak with the consultant right

---

away and before seeing her son. There being no consultant available, I agreed to see her in a few moments. The young man had overheard this conversation and nodded his agreement for me to speak with his mother.

As I walked out of the ward towards the waiting room, the ward sister told me some more of the story. She said that the man had been admitted by 'blue light' ambulance at 4 AM. He had been found alone and asleep in a side street. He smelt strongly of alcohol and urine and had been covered in blood. He was rather abusive to the staff and had been warned of the 'zero-tolerance' policy for staff abuse in the department. He had adamantly refused to let contact be made with friends or relatives. He had been taken into the majors' resuscitation area where a drip had been put up and his blood pressure and pulse taken. After his arm was sutured, he was put in a ward bed for observation for the rest of the night. He had slept soundly until we reviewed him on the ward round.

We entered the visitor's room and found a woman of about 45 and a man, presumably a close relative, comforting her. She had obviously been crying but stood up as we entered and thanked us for seeing her. The man remained silent holding her hand. As we all sat down she began her side of the story ... ...

Some questions to consider as you read this chapter
- What do we mean by 'the context of the case'?
- Why does the context (beyond the immediate and obvious) matter?
- What cues should direct us to explore the context further?
- What elements of the context should we take account of?
- Who is part of the context of a case?
- How does the kind of person you are influence your management of a case?

INTRODUCTION

This chapter considers the first of our invisibles, which is the importance of thoroughly exploring the implicit and tacit context of a patient's case. In addition to the opening scenario, the chapter is divided into five sections. The first sets the scene by exploring the need for the doctor to be aware of and sensitive to the richness of detail of the patient case. The second introduces the significance within this of the particular context in which the doctor first meets the patient. The first heuristic is then introduced in the third section. The fourth section offers three resources, each designed to facilitate the further exploration of these ideas.

Finally, a follow-up scenario is offered to the trainee doctor's story that prefaces this chapter, and the reader is invited to explore the whole scenario in the light of the content of the chapter. Some suggested further reading is appended to the end of the chapter.

THE NEED FOR SENSITIVITY TO THE RICHNESS OF THE PATIENT CASE

The story that prefaces this chapter is at several removes from the original event. It is no longer simply the patient's story, and it is not told by the patient. Rather it has become a trainee's story – a trainee who has 'inherited' the patient on a Sunday morning from a colleague who first dealt with the patient during Saturday night. This trainee meets both patient and a version of his story 'the morning after' (a phrase that has the nuance of alcoholism about it).

This story is extended at the end of this chapter, and we shall see as events unfold that it is far less simple than at first appears. Indeed, even in the opening part, the story quickly begins to take on some complexity as further narrators join in. The complexity, however, should not have been unexpected, and there is enough detail available already in the story so far to indicate this. But the trainee who was present when the patient arrived in A & E was seduced by appearances and too easily accepted some apparently obvious implications. These had been crystallized by time and circumstances into a diagnosis and management that was so routine that the doctors had stopped looking at it.

At first meeting the patient and as a natural part of taking the patient's history and listening to the patient narrative, doctors always obtain and record the basic context of that case. And those details are carefully re-presented to colleagues as the patient is handed over to the next shift. This handover is crucial, and it has two aspects that repay further exploration. The first is in respect of the patient case; the second is in respect of the role of the doctor within that case (and his/her awareness of that role).

The patient case

A close look at the *content* of the 'patient history' and the traditional language in which it is captured and conveyed reveals that a considerable element of ritual is involved, together with a seriously limited view of what might constitute the significant contextual details. Further, as with any handing on of 'facts' from one person to another, there are multiple points at which interpretation of the details rather than an exact repetition of them can occur. Here, the 'objective truth' of science imperceptibly gives way to the subjective interpretation of the humanities.

Case presentation is full of ritual elements. These consist of the patient's age, gender, family details, significant recent history and immediate cause of hospitalization. These are the formulaic responses to the question: Why is this patient here, with this problem, now? These are the basics that all doctors have been taught to obtain, record and hand on. But beneath this apparently simple set of facts may simmer unnoticed details that a more sensitive (and experienced) eye and ear would have recognized. These can sometimes transform the entire interpretation of the case. This is what separates the novice from the expert doctor.

Given what we know of the 'complexity, unpredictability, paradox and uncertainty' (Fish and Coles, 2005, p. 105) of medical practice generally, it seems somewhat naive to assume that the details emerging from the basic handover rituals are always sufficient. Indeed, we would argue that, by definition, any case selected for learning doctors' more detailed scrutiny would be one worthy of extended investigation, especially in respect of the contextualizing details.

Experienced doctors have learnt to seek and to pick up clues about whether a more detailed context is needed, and/or they are intuitive about there being more to the case than meets the eye. Learning doctors, in a hurry to move into diagnosis and patient management, can fail to take account of the full contextual details. They need to remember that appearances can be deceptive and that their awareness needs to be at its sharpest at the point of first meeting the patient.

The doctor as interpreter of the patient's case

On first engaging with a patient, any doctor becomes a learner about both the patient and about the patient's case, and an interpreter and conveyer onwards of the significant details of it.

This is a far more sophisticated and significant process than is sometimes recognized. At first meeting (particularly with new patients) in their speedy sizing up of the patient and their rapid synthesizing of the patient's case, doctors are engaged in far more than they often realize. They use all their senses both to collect information and to process that information – not only 'scientifically' but, more importantly, '*unscientifically*'!

Iona Heath (herself a doctor) importantly draws attention to the complexity of what doctors have to synthesize, and what they bring to this, in the following (Heath, 1998, p. 87):

'If the full potential of the patient's story is to be realized, [the] doctor ... needs to be willing to listen, to hear and to be literate at many different levels.'

Heath goes on to enumerate those levels as medical literacy, physical literacy, emotional literacy and cultural literacy. This list is a sharp reminder of how much more there is in this process than simply 'doing medicine'. She expands this as follows.

Medical literacy ensures that when the patient has a disease for which medicine offers effective treatment, the pattern of the patient's symptoms will be recognized and appropriate action taken. Physical literacy makes use of the doctor's subjective awareness of his or her own body, combined with his or her objective knowledge of the body as a physical specimen. This combination underpins the empathic interpretation of the patient's symptoms that lies at the root of diagnosis. Emotional literacy allows the doctor to acknowledge and witness the patient's suffering and pain and help in the struggle to find a way forward. Cultural literacy enriches the search for meaning with examples of the way others have made healing sense of the same sorts of hurt and pain (Heath, 1998, p. 87).

To this list we would add – at its very beginning – the recognition of the role of meaning-making in medicine (an understanding of processes of interpretation and the significance of nuance), because in all of Heath's important 'literacies' the doctor is concerned much less with science and 'objective' fact (if there is such a thing) than with *interpretation*. As Greenhalgh and Hurwitz (1998a, p. 6) say:

> 'When doctors take a medical history we inevitably act as ethnographers, historians and biographers, requiring to understand aspects of personhood, personality, social and psychological functioning as well as biological and physical phenomena.
>
> Thus patient's narratives provide us with far more than factual information of the kind that might be more efficiently obtained [through] electronic smart cards ....
>
> The narrative provides meaning, context and perspective for the patient's predicament. It defines how and why and in what way he or she is ill. It offers in short, a possibility of *understanding* which cannot be arrived at by any other means.'

But as we shall argue throughout this book, the holistic understanding of the patient requires a holistic response from the doctor. An awareness of the doctor's part in the patient's story is the starting point for this.

This is because – whether they take account of it or not – doctors are not only 'outside agents', but are also, from their first meeting with the patient, *inside the patient's story*. They are a part of the very context that they are trying to understand.

The importance of context: Introducing Heuristic 1

Every case is context-specific. Doctors' recognition and interpretation of the context in which they meet the patient and hear the patient's story, then, is crucial in understanding the case and in setting the whole course of both diagnosis and management. Thus, the significance of context and the role it plays cannot be overemphasized.

But the context involves more than the patient, other carers (friends, family and other healthcare colleagues) and the setting in which they are met. It importantly includes the doctor him- or herself, and what they bring to that first meeting. Indeed, the manifestation of the patient's problem(s) is perceived through the lenses the doctor brings up to it, and the formulation of the problem (and all that follows from it in the way of diagnosis and management) is filtered through the doctor's interpretive processes.

Thus the doctor is not only the key meaning-maker of the patient's case (engaging in interpretation at all points), but is also a factor *within* the very context in which they meet the patient, contributing a whole dimension to that very event. Indeed, doctors' subsequent decisions and actions in respect of a patient are only intelligible (explicable and defendable) by reference to their own understanding and interpretation of the case.

So, we argue, patient cases need to be more thoroughly contextualized by learning doctors than they usually are. By exploring the context of the case in detail as the starting point for management, doctors can become more aware of and develop greater sensitivity to the nuances of meaning and the complexity of interpretation that they (often unwittingly) engage in as they treat patients. Whilst this is already done in broad terms in discussion with peers or supervisor, this rarely allows enough time to explore the subtleties of the case. By contrast, writing about the case helps the development of insight, imagination, awareness and sensitivity to the individuality of patient cases.

We offer Heuristic 1 and the subsequent learning resources to help doctors in thinking these cases through.

HEURISTIC 1: THE PICTURE (AFTER MONET'S *WOMAN SITTING UNDER WILLOWS*)

The picture provided by this heuristic represents an invitation to explore contextual evidence in relation to a common human event but outside a patient case. This allows us to point up – and we hope to encourage readers to remember – the considerable range of human issues that may need to be fleshed out before the patient's story can be fully appreciated, before the doctor's understanding of it can be wholly established, and before a treatment plan can begin to emerge.

Accordingly, the reader is invited to take a few minutes to consider the picture shown in Figure 4.1, to identify the key contextual details of the entire scene, to answer the questions that appear around the picture, and to ascertain whether or not this is, as it seems to be, a picture of a picnic.

Our picture is deliberately based on a familiar and famous painting, which is itself part of a series of paintings by Monet, because we believe that it will be more memorable for seeming familiar. We hope thereby that doctors will call it to mind readily both within the clinical setting and when reflecting upon it afterwards. We have produced this scene as a line drawing and added some elements that were not in the original in order to emphasize the complexity and ambiguities that are so often part of a scenario, especially when we meet it for the first time.

There's always more than meets the eye

In responding to the invitation to consider the details of the depicted scene, readers will quickly establish that all that can be hazarded in respect of the context of the event depicted is interpretation rather than concrete fact. There are no clear facts about why the people in the picture have met. Implication rather than explicit evidence is all that exists. Various elements conjoin together to imply that this is a picnic, but it could be a meeting for a quite other purpose. Intuition rather than logic suggests that they have come from the nearby town, but there seems no clear reason for them to have done so on this occasion. Further, from the presentation of the picture, there is no real way of being sure what are the

What details can you provide about the *context* of what is happening in this picture:

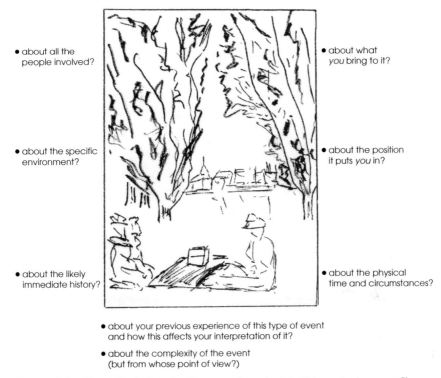

● about all the
people involved?

● about what
you bring to it?

● about the specific
environment?

● about the position
it puts *you* in?

● about the likely
immediate history?

● about the physical
time and circumstances?

● about your previous experience of this type of event
and how this affects your interpretation of it?

● about the complexity of the event
(but from whose point of view?)

Figure 4.1   Heuristic 1: the significance of context (Is this a picnic or not?).

salient facts and what are random elements connected either by the imagination of the painter or the fleeting recognition of something personally familiar to the observer. Perhaps we should not rush so readily to assumption. This could be a picnic (and all three people could be meeting for pleasure), but equally it could be a meeting between criminals to share the loot or the hasty repast of a group of people on the run for some reason. Some of the visible 'facts' of the case would fit any one of these explanations. None of these explanations fits all the facts.

We are now left with the question for the learning doctor: What details can you now provide about the context of your meeting(s) with the patient in respect of a specific case? The following learning resources are designed to help with this.

THREE LEARNING RESOURCES FOR USE IN EXPLORING CONTEXT

Resource 4.1: Situational or contextual analysis of a case

Resource 4.1 provides some questions that should help the detailed contextual-ization of the given case. This is based broadly on the ideas of Malcolm Skilbeck,

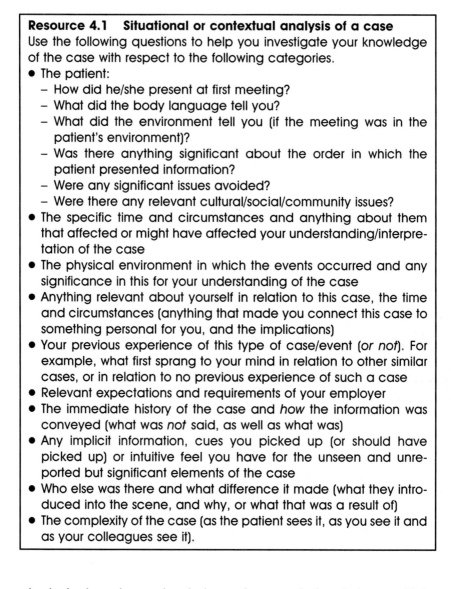

Resource 4.1   Situational or contextual analysis of a case
Use the following questions to help you investigate your knowledge of the case with respect to the following categories.
- The patient:
  - How did he/she present at first meeting?
  - What did the body language tell you?
  - What did the environment tell you (if the meeting was in the patient's environment)?
  - Was there anything significant about the order in which the patient presented information?
  - Were any significant issues avoided?
  - Were there any relevant cultural/social/community issues?
- The specific time and circumstances and anything about them that affected or might have affected your understanding/interpretation of the case
- The physical environment in which the events occurred and any significance in this for your understanding of the case
- Anything relevant about yourself in relation to this case, the time and circumstances (anything that made you connect this case to something personal for you, and the implications)
- Your previous experience of this type of case/event (*or not*). For example, what first sprang to your mind in relation to other similar cases, or in relation to no previous experience of such a case
- Relevant expectations and requirements of your employer
- The immediate history of the case and *how* the information was conveyed (what was *not* said, as well as what was)
- Any implicit information, cues you picked up (or should have picked up) or intuitive feel you have for the unseen and unreported but significant elements of the case
- Who else was there and what difference it made (what they introduced into the scene, and why, or what that was a result of)
- The complexity of the case (as the patient sees it, as you see it and as your colleagues see it).

who, in the days when teachers had control over curriculum design, provided a set of questions to support what he called 'a situational analysis' of the teaching context.

Of course, not every question will have equal importance in every case. These ideas are to be used flexibly and as needed. We do believe, however, that collecting a portfolio of cases that have been examined in this detail will not only provide learning doctors and their teachers with evidence of progress in developing awareness of and sensitivity to the context, but will also help to improve the picking up of important cues in practice itself. However there is more to it than this.

We have argued that the doctor is both a part of the context of the situation in which the patient presents him or herself and the key interpreter of that context and that presentation. Accordingly, Resource 4.2, which follows, offers details of how the doctor can explore the kind of person that he/she brings to the case, while Resource 4.3 then offers some further issues for consideration about the processes of interpretation.

Resource 4.2: The kind of person the doctor is and aspires to be

Clearly, as a doctor meeting, diagnosing and managing patients, it is not just what one knows that matters, but the kind of person one is. The person one is affects how one uses the knowledge and skills one has. (If one is interested only in the science of the disease and not how it affects the patient, this is different from seeing the patient as the person who has the disease.) This is why the specific qualities that the doctor as a person brings to the context of a specific case significantly affect the care of the patient and are significant in the relationship established with the patient. (This latter point deserves a more detailed exploration, which we provide for in Chapter 9.)

Doctors then, need ways of refining their awareness of both what they as a person bring to the patient case and that affect their interpretations of it, and how they might wish to develop and refine these key personal qualities.

One way that learning doctors can achieve this is by the rigorous investigation of their *feelings, expectations, assumptions, beliefs, intuitions ('sixth sense'), attitudes, insight/imagination* and *personal values*, as illuminated by their conduct in a specific patient case.

What are values?

Values are those abiding and long-cherished views about what we see as enduringly worthwhile and important. For all of us who practise in a profession, values shape both our view of the world at large and our professional practice specifically. They profoundly influence how we seek to conduct ourselves. They are tacit, lying deep beneath the surface elements of practice, but they are highly significant as the key 'drivers' of how we conduct ourselves in practice.

Values are by definition matters of contention, since they are often not shared by others in our working environment, or even across professions. Everyone who works in healthcare lives at the centre of a web of complex, but subtle and largely invisible pressures which arise from the differing values endemic to clinical practice and its management (de Cossart and Fish, 2005, p. 20). Indeed, because values are rarely directly discussed, (so that colleagues do not recognize their differences as being values-based), the pressures that arise from them are not traced to source, and thus become puzzling as well as frustrating.

Complex though values are, they are central and fundamental to the nature of professional practice and its expertise, and we therefore have to begin any attempt to understand and develop that practice, by exploring them.

Developing the Wise Doctor

Practitioners rarely talk or write directly about their values, but, despite this, what they do, know and think speaks volumes in respect of what they believe is important. Indeed, ironically, that which practitioners take for granted, and over-look (because it is so much a natural part of their practice), is often very visible to patients and other colleagues who observe them (Fish and Coles, 2005, pp. 81–2).

The iceberg of practice

We have in the past used the following picture of the iceberg – first developed by Fish and Coles (1998) – to remind us of most of these tacit elements that lie deep beneath the surface of practice. This originally contained *experience, knowledge, feelings, expectations, assumptions, beliefs, attitudes,* and *personal values,* but we have now removed *experience* and *knowledge* because they are attended to in Chapter 6, and have added *intuitions ('sixth sense')* and *insight/imagination* (which, though also referred to in Chapter 6, are important to consider here).

By 'beliefs' in the above, we do not only mean spiritual/religious beliefs but also broader beliefs about self and life. For example, does the doctor think of

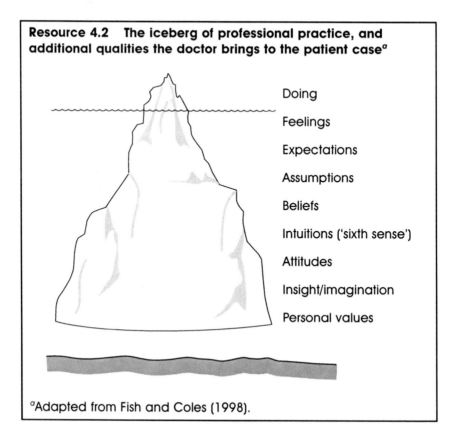

Resource 4.2   The iceberg of professional practice, and additional qualities the doctor brings to the patient case[a]

Doing

Feelings

Expectations

Assumptions

Beliefs

Intuitions ('sixth sense')

Attitudes

Insight/imagination

Personal values

[a]Adapted from Fish and Coles (1998).

cases or patients; does he/she see the disease having the patient or the patient having the disease? Beliefs are stronger than expectations or assumptions.

Some further comments

In respect of all this, teachers and assessors need to think about the traditional emphasis in postgraduate medicine on 'knowledge and skills' and what this does to the other important elements of patient care. They also need to be sensitive to the influence they have (both explicitly and as models) on the doctors in their care. For example, what teachers expect junior doctors to know will influence what they learn. What is more, the teacher's expectations and attitudes will influence the learner's view of the balance that should exist between scientific and humanistic elements of practice.

Further, in the busy clinical environment, the teacher who recognizes a young doctor's good rapport with patients should praise it and as a result provide an encouraging basis for them to develop their knowledge and skills of the disease, rather than highlighting and emphasizing their lack of knowledge of the range of elements of the disease, thereby demotivating them.

The following resource offers a non-medical but nonetheless relevant example of the importance of interpretation.

Resource 4.3: The 'Three Mile Island' incident

Doctors who are still caught up in positivistic attitudes to 'objective truth' would regard the significance of interpretation as unscientific. As Greenhalgh and Hurwitz (1998a, p. 10) point out:

> 'The study of interpretation (the discernment of meaning) is a central concern of philosophers and linguists, but it is a concept with which doctors and … scientists are often unfamiliar, and hence uncomfortable. We recognize, but cannot elucidate with our familiar scientific tools, the meaning the narrative gives to sequences of events [and we would add: and also to their context], a meaning that … asserts a particular human significance, whether symbolic, biographical or biological.'

Resource 4.3 provides a story that readers may like to relate to medicine, either as they read it or subsequently. In so doing, they might also ponder the words of Asher, quoted in Greenhalgh and Hurwitz (1998a, p. 9) as graphic in drawing doctor's attention to the dangerous tendency of clinicians to see the expected and unconsciously to dismiss the anomalous. They say of this:

> 'We have to be aware of this suppressive faculty which, by producing selective deafness, selective blindness and other sense rejections, can easily suppress the significant and the relevant …'

Donald Schön, the author and teacher who established the importance of the professional as reflective practitioner, told the following story in Schön (1987a), and also offered it the same year as part of a lecture at the Royal Society of Arts in

Resource 4.3   The 'Three Mile Island' incident

When the nuclear plant at Three Mile Island began to show signs of meltdown, operators were alerted to the problem by the ringing of one alarm only. This they initially interpreted as needing attention, but as not serious. However, in fact, multiple errors had occurred. Complicating this, a light designed to indicate a serious malfunction was covered by a maintenance tag, and nobody saw it.

The staff took action to deal with what they thought was an isolated problem. But this, in fact, made the overall situation much worse. It was then that the problem escalated sharply. In looking into the incident later, observers reported that staff suddenly saw across the whole main control panel a 'Christmas Tree' of alarm lights. None had experienced anything like this before. There was no guidance about this level of danger in their book of procedures. The staff became helpless in the face of near disaster.

Schön's observation was that the operators were not prepared for what he called 'surprises' – indeed, that the management of the reactor had attempted 'to avoid surprise, employing for this purpose a full panoply of measures, systems of control, targets and systems of reward and punishment to reinforce measures' (Schön, 1987b, p. 227).

He locates the failure of the operators to respond appropriately to the complex problems they faced in what he calls 'proceduralization and control'. He notes that 'surprises' will occur and are not eliminated by having carefully written procedures, because those protocols were drawn up to cope with previous problems rather than completely new ones. He comments that one consequence of proceduralization is that 'people get to be very good ... at not noticing surprise' and systematically avoid attending to information – which he calls 'weird' or 'junk' data – that would cause uncertainty.

A further problem of proceduralization, according to Schön, is the development of multiple systems of control. As he says: 'When things go wrong in spite of the fact that we multiply procedures to keep them from happening, the response is to increase and improve the procedures. So after Three Mile Island, investigators proposed to expand the book of procedures.' However, he comments (Schön, 1987b, p. 228):

'When we adopt such remedies we drive out wisdom, artistry and "feel for phenomena", all of which depend on judgment. We produce a world of increased routinization and control and dubious achievement with respect to the disasters we wish to avoid. ... For practitioners, the cumulative effect of such remedies is [that] artistry, wisdom, judgement, feel for materials, all of which depend upon discretionary freedom, get progressively squeezed out of practice as control and procedures are multiplied in order to avoid unpleasant surprises.'

He notes on the same page that 'managers try to control subordinates by imposing measures of performance on them; and subordinates find ways to meet the letter of the measures without meeting their spirit'. He suggests that, as a result, 'the system of the organization becomes undiscussable ...'. He adds ironically: 'Moreover, undiscussability turns readily to indescribability. Without discussion, we do not practise describing what goes on; and since we cannot describe it, we would not be very good at discussing it even if we were willing to do so' (Schön, 1987, p. 228).

London (Schön 1987b). In this story, he analyses a near disaster that occurred at a nuclear reactor in New Jersey in the mid-1970s as a means of highlighting the danger of merely relying on quick sifting of sensory information.

Readers might like to provide examples from, or to analyze in detail, a whole case in which they later became aware that they had exercised selective deafness, selective blindness and other sense rejections, or otherwise overlooked the significant and the relevant.

They might also like to list examples of the cues that needed to be attended to in order to avoid the serious misinterpretation of a case or aspects of it.

FOLLOW-UP SCENARIO: 'THERE'S MORE THAN MEETS THE EYE'

The following details offer further perspectives on the story with which this chapter began.

The mother's story
After shaking hands with us, the patient's mother began:

'David has a brain tumour, which was diagnosed about three months ago. He had been having 'funny turns', especially after drinking, over about the last six months – long before the diagnosis. The doctors think the epilepsy was induced by alcohol. He is booked for surgery in two weeks time at the Neurosciences Centre under Mr Phelps. They have told him that it may leave him with some paralysis in his arm and had offered him some counselling support, which he had refused. He had not touched alcohol since the diagnosis. Yesterday he had gone to his friend's in the morning. They were planning a day in the town followed by a meal and he had said that he would probably stay over at his friend's, so not to expect him home.

'This morning at 8 AM his friend called to make sure that he had got home OK. He was surprised to find he was not there, as he had left his friends in town in the early evening saying that he had to get out of the pub as he felt hemmed in, and that he was going home. They had not seen him since and had assumed that he had gone home.

'David has been rather morose for the past week and we have been keen that he should enjoy himself with his friends. He had been reluctant to talk about his problem. We wanted to talk to you before seeing him so that we could be prepared to know how we should help him and would very much appreciate your advice, especially to try and get him to agree to see the support counsellor in the "neuro" department. I hope that he is going to be alright', she finished rather breathlessly.

I then explained that David was OK and the cut on his arm was very superficial. I said that we should go and see him together and that we should discuss the planned surgery and the importance of him receiving support to deal with a very threatening problem. The nurse suggested bringing David to us and went off to fetch him. He came in, and a very tearful reunion took place. Later he agreed to meet the 'neuro' team and an appointment was arranged for the next day. He went home with his parents.

Reflective diary note by the night SpR from this scenario

◆ Busy night on Saturday; a lot of complex trauma and great challenges to my ability to triage. Most of the major cases went OK. Really enjoyed it.

◆ Bit concerned about boy found unconscious in the street though. Did not get to the point there.

◆ Did not really go into depth of the case as it seemed pretty straightforward.

◆ Should have queried the incontinence more. Didn't listen to my alarm bells or perhaps they were not ringing!

◆ Was a bit hard on the alcohol in retrospect. We had just been to the lecture on zero tolerance and I guess we were trying it out!!! Not a very appropriate start ... must put things into perspective.

◆ Should have got the nurses to press him more for contacts but they were so busy and I had my mind on other things ... which I thought were more important ... and were certainly more 'exciting' and relevant to my aim of managing major trauma. Must try and not get seduced by things as I might miss very important things.

◆ Think I dropped SpR 2 in it. Feel bad about that – need to talk to him. Thank God he is a thoughtful person.

NEED TO THINK ABOUT
My ability to become fully engaged in one thing and miss other things of importance.

My need to temper my enthusiasm for the 'zero tolerance' matter by finding out the true facts.

My need to take an overall view of the scene rather than get stuck in one corner of it and relying on others to manage the more mundane!

MUST TALK TO JIM!

Commentary

The patient had arrived at a busy time in A & E. Staff abuse as a result of alcohol was high on everyone's agenda. Certain assumptions relating to the patient's presentation and demeanour were therefore made. These were reinforced by his behaviour and uncommunicative responses. Too many assumptions were made, based on too few observations. No one checked out the original interpretation of the case – not even on the ward round the next morning. Someone should have sat down and talked with the patient.

Thus the things we wish doctors to learn in considering the context, and by using the heuristic and these resources, is how they can best deal sensitively with the interpretation of cases with which they are involved and which will vary in their complexity.

FURTHER READING

Joyce J (1998) A Painful Case. In: *The Dubliners*. London: Penguin [originally published 1914].

Hurwitz B (1998) The wounded Storyteller: narrative strands in medical negligence. In: Greenhalgh T, Hurwitz B, eds. *Narrative Based Medicine: Dialogue and Discourse in Clinical Practice*. London: BMJ Books.

5

Exploring the doctor's professionalism: Prompted by Heuristic 2

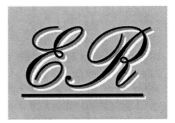

OPENING SCENARIO

You are invited to read this chapter with the following scenario in mind:

The kind of professional you think you are ...

Scene: the consultant's office

Consultant (Cons): I was on ward XZ with the manager yesterday and observed from a distance your ward round with the F2 doctor, medical student and staff nurse. There seemed to be some disquiet after you had left Mrs Smith. ... Would you like to tell me about how *you* view what happened there?

Specialist Registrar (SpR): Well ... I was doing my usual daily ward round and had just told that patient in bed six ... Mrs ... um, Smith ... that she could go home. She'd been in hospital two weeks with cellulitis of her leg and is now on oral antibiotics. ... She ... she *was* worried about when she would be seen again ... um, ... I left the nurse to sort all that out. ... we were running late because of the audit meeting and needed to get on ...

Cons: Yes, I know about your clinical responsibilities here. But what I am trying to understand now is more about you. What qualities in a doctor do you think would matter most to Mrs Smith ... well, and to patients and colleagues generally. ... For example, what do you think your colleagues learnt yesterday about being a doctor ... being a professional ... about you as a doctor?

SpR: Well ... um ... they certainly learned about how clinical life is busy and how you need to keep up a good pace on the ward round. ... And that I am able to do it.

Cons: Yes, but being a good doctor is not just about being efficient is it? ... What else is involved?

SpR: Oh I see. I suppose you are testing my communication skills.

Cons: Well no, I'm not trying to test anything. I'm inviting you to explore some ideas with me. You are training to be a senior professional in medicine ... so I genuinely want you to talk with me about what you understand about your wider responsibilities to patients and other members of the team in which you work. What would other members of the team have learned yesterday *about you as a doctor*?

SpR: Well, ... um ... that I am efficient and can get through the work.

Cons: You are right. But what kind of consultant do you aspire to be? Don't you think good doctors need other important qualities to complement that efficiency?

SpR: I suppose so ... but I do feel strongly that my responsibilities are first towards my patients and getting through the work.

Cons: Yes – but what else does the word 'responsibilities' here imply? What is actually involved in being a good professional? It isn't just skills and efficiency is it? ... Isn't there something more?

SpR: Yes ... Probably ... but it's hard to put into words ... We talked about that a bit at medical school ... but somehow it's different now ... Can I think about this some more and come back to you?

Cons: Yes. ... Good ... I would suggest that you use Heuristic 2 to help you create some points for us to discuss your professionalism and conduct in relation to the case of Mrs Smith. Don't use it to label yourself into one of its categories, use it to help you think. Then, using Resource 5.1 here [offers resource] construct a statement of your professional values in general. Shall we meet again on Friday at 4.30 PM then? Good luck.

Some questions to consider as you read this chapter
- What kind of doctor are you?
- Why does it matter what kind of doctor you are?
- To whom does it matter?
- What kind of doctor do you think others see you as?
- What kind of doctor are you seeking to become?

- Why do you need to continue to consider the kind of doctor you want to be?
- How would you explain your key professional values and why they matter?
- How would you express your professional vision and when might you need to do so?
- How does this affect your critique of your own professional development?
- How does it allow you to develop as an active partner in the development of both healthcare and education?

INTRODUCTION

This chapter begins by outlining the importance of professionalism generally and the reasons why learning doctors need to continue to keep their professionalism under review. It then offers Heuristic 2, which prompts (in relation to a given case) an exploration of those features of practice that demonstrate the qualities of a restricted or extended professional. This heuristic is followed by four sets of supporting materials that are provided as resources to help teachers and learners to explore these matters further – firstly at an individual level, and secondly in profession-wide terms. At all points, ideas for using these resources educationally are also provided.

Heuristic 2 invites doctors to consider their conduct (and therefore their professionalism) in relation to a given case or – better – in relation to several cases. Resource 5.1 introduces two significant subcategories: 'espoused professional values', which enshrine *aspirations* about how to conduct oneself in the clinical setting, and 'values-in-use', which draw on how one actually conducts oneself across clinical settings, and which allow a professional to tease out the values that actually lie under their practice as it is 'lived'. This will enable the doctor to begin to generalize about and begin to shape and organize how they articulate their own professionalism.

Resource 5.2 is also focused on the individual's professional values, and offers a list of ideas to facilitate an exploration of what is involved in being a member of a profession as opposed to merely 'behaving professionally'. This will enable learning doctors to refine the language and ideas in which they express their professionalism. Suggestions are then made about developing in writing, keeping updated and using, in various contexts, a carefully articulated statement of one's professional vision or philosophy.

Resources 5.3 and 5.4 widen the focus to consider the values of a profession as a whole. Resource 5.3 offers a chart of two differing visions of professional practice and highlights their underlying values. Resource 5.4 provides details of the official professional values of medicine as a whole. Doctors are encouraged to consider how these relate to their own values and to those of other professions represented within the multidisciplinary team.

The final scenario then offers a professional conversation, together with an appreciation of it, that extends the opening scenario and shows how some of these ideas might be developed educationally between supervisor and supervisee. Finally, further reading is provided that will enable this thinking to be extended further.

THE IMPORTANCE OF PROFESSIONALISM

Professionalism is an aspect of practice that is assessed in all doctors at all points from the Foundation Years to the end of specialty training. It is significant in shaping good relationships with all heathcare colleagues. It is recognized by the sick as central to the quality of their care, and is a crucial element in patients' attitudes to their doctors. The recent Royal College of Physicians (RCP) report on the importance of medical professionalism sees it as underpinning the trust that the public has in doctors and states: 'Patients certainly understand the meaning of poor professionalism and associate it with poor medical care.' It continues: 'The public is well aware that an absence of professionalism is harmful to their interests' (RCP, 2005, p. xi). Professionalism, then, is also a critical factor in the consideration of clinical governance and in medicolegal situations.

But what is meant by professionalism? All practising doctors believe that they know what is involved in being a professional in today's NHS. However, the professional ideals, aspirations and values that drive practice are far from easy to unearth and express clearly. As a consequence, doctors have until recently mostly been content to leave them as implicit or even tacit. However, it has now become clear to the medical profession that it is vital that 'doctors must be clearer about what they do and how and why they do it' (RCP, 2005, p. xi).

It is therefore important that doctors in training be enabled to explore, make explicit, defend and critique the key principles and values to which they aspire and which they intend to use to shape their working lives as medical practitioners. Further, it is equally important that they then be helped to find the courage both to explore their practice in terms of these values (identifying where their aspirations do not match their actual conduct), and explore their intended values in terms of what medical practice currently allows or encourages. The gap between one's espoused values and those that are found in one's practice, as well as the gap between how one is permitted to practice and the values one wishes to espouse, will indicate aspects of one's conduct and one's views about professionalism, all of which need in some way to be worked upon critically.

Currently, there are no guidelines to support how this important topic could be taught, learnt and assessed. Accordingly, this chapter, from opening to closing scenario, sets out to offer some starting points and ideas and prompt some ways of thinking about, and finding the language in which to express, these matters.

In the scenario that begins this chapter, we can see that the consultant has picked up from observation that the SpR's conduct in a clinical setting had caused unease both in a patient and amongst colleagues. In their subsequent private meeting after this incident, the consultant eschews the traditional teaching session in which 'feedback' on the SpR's performance would normally be offered (and where the learner would feel they were in an assessment session) in favour of a more adventurous teaching mode. Rather than telling the learner, the consultant engages (motivates) the SpR to explore her own understanding of her professionalism in relation to the specific piece of practice in question. The consultant does so by providing stimulating resources and by asking the SpR to consider the clinical scenario and explore her priorities within it ready to discuss them, and then to commit to paper a written version of her more general aspirations for her future professional conduct. As we said in Chapter 3, a learner who engages only in discussion, where there is no permanent record of achievement, may be falsely persuaded at the end of it that either he/she has made no progress or worse, that he/she really knew it all already. A written version is able to be reviewed later as ideas are challenged and grow. Such a review demonstrates and provides unequivocal evidence of progress, or lack of it.

We see clearly from the dialogue in the opening scenario that, at the start of this educational sequence, the SpR was not at all alert to the issues that needed to be explored, did not pick up the invitation to talk about her qualities as a doctor, could not easily shed the notion that she was being tested, and kept 'ducking out' of the challenge being offered and back into traditional, even ritualistic talk, about ward rounds. At first, on the SpR's part, this looks like deliberate obtuseness, defensiveness or even ignorance of the real issues. This (importantly) causes the consultant, gently but firmly to press home her agenda.

As the consultant continues to prompt and press the issues about professionalism, the SpR begins to gain insight into what is being asked, remembers earlier discussions, and herself recognizes the need to think more deeply about the ideas and to find a way of talking about them. This is the breakthrough the consultant is seeking. Praise is then offered, supportive materials are provided, a written task is offered and a new meeting is agreed. It should be noted that the task set is carefully designed not as a formal assessment, but to provide the basis for the next discussion, to capture evidence of where the learner has started, as a baseline for this discussion, and to enable continuity of theme and thus of education. Progress can now be made – as we shall see at the end of the chapter.

The supportive materials that were offered by the consultant in the opening scenario now follow as Heuristic 2 and Resource 5.1.

HEURISTIC 2 AND ITS USES

The design of this prompt has been based on ideas developed in 1974 by Eric Hoyle, which he originally offered, at the point when teaching became an all-graduate profession, to help teachers to consider the quality of their professional commitment. It is designed to be used in respect of one's conduct within a specific case or cases, rather than at the level of generality. Further, it is intended as a set of ideas that, like a springboard, free readers to explore their own conduct. Its intention is to encourage practitioners to recognize and move on from a narrow to a broader view of what is involved in being a professional. See Figure 5.1.

How to use Heuristic 2

A simplistic approach to using this heuristic should be avoided. For example, it should not be assumed that the restricted professional is always the new member

EXTENDED PROFESSIONAL	RESTRICTED PROFESSIONAL
Own clinical skills derived from relating experience and theory of all kinds, through rigorous reflection	Own clinical skills are derived from experience. Only interested in survival and simply getting on with the job
Perspectives embrace wider social context and later times (long- as well as short-term goals are of concern)	Perspectives restricted to 'what happens now' (only short-term goals are of concern)
Sees clinical practice as complex, intriguing, problematic, driven by values, beliefs, assumptions and needing to be seated in a professional philosophy	Sees clinical practice as technical procedures that merit little educational interest because learning them only requires plenty of repetition
Clinical events seen in relation to social policies and wider goals	Clinical events are seen in isolation each from the other and from any wider perspectives
Own clinical methods and processes compared with those of colleagues and with reports of other practice	Introspective about own clinical methods and processes
Value placed on professional collaboration within and beyond own profession	High value placed on own autonomy
High value on the whole range of professional activities – locally, within hospital Trust, and nationally	Limited involvement in all but direct clinical activities
Frequent reading of a wide range of literature relevant to professional practice generally	Infrequent reading of a range of literature beyond immediate clinical specialty
Involvement in professional development at a range of levels (personal and collegiate)	Least possible involvement in professional development (and only at personal level)

Figure 5.1 Heuristic 2: the kind of professional you are (to be used in exploring a specific case) (adapted from de Cossart and Fish, 2005, p. 112).

of the profession and the extended professional the more experienced member. Young and new doctors might be extended professionals, while older but narrower thinking staff might be restricted ones. Further, it may be possible to find oneself somewhere on a continuum between these two polarities, or to realize that one is restricted in respect of one category and extended in respect of another. The important ideas to explore, prompted by this heuristic, relate to the views professionals hold of what is (or should be) involved in their daily conduct as professionals. By conduct here, we mean actions together with what drives those actions.

We believe that this heuristic puts flesh on the ideas about what it is to be a professional, as first expressed by Professor Mike Golby, who said that professionals are 'persons who seek a broad understanding of their practice, paying attention not only to their developing competence, but also to the fundamental purposes and values that underpin their work' (Golby, 1993, p. 5).

Accordingly, we would advise readers to use this prompt to ask themselves how they see the fundamental purposes and values of their professional work. This can best be done by taking a case example and exploring one's own professionalism in respect of it. This will inevitably lead to the identification of some key personal professional values. The following resource may be of help in teasing these out.

RESOURCE 5.1: IDEAS FOR EXPLORING PROFESSIONAL VALUES

The following points offer ideas on what professional values are and thus provide a means for beginning to explore them.

Resource 5.1   Exploring professional values

SOME POINTS TO CONSIDER

- Your professional values are how you consistently see the world in which you engage in professional practice, and what you prioritize in your professional life. Your professional values are what drive your professional actions, attitudes, thoughts and beliefs
- Your values exist well before you become conscious of them, and, whether you are aware of them or not, they are evident to and have a profound effect on others
- Your professional values shape how you conduct yourself in the clinical setting. And your conduct in the clinical setting reveals your values to all those you work with (colleagues and patients)
- Your values will affect how you learn and what you gain from the learning opportunities available to you

---

- Sometimes our *actions* reveal values that are different from those we would *say* we held. (We might claim to value the patient's views, but how we behave towards them might tell them that we do not!) Here there is a gap between our espoused values (values we claim to hold) and our values in use (values that emerge from our practice)
- Whilst our espoused values and our values in use are in harmony, there is no conflict, but this is rare, and something to strive for rather than something we can easily attain. When we recognize such a gap, it is always worth exploring further both our practice and our values
- When we do so, we may discover values that we should act upon but which we have not prioritized and which therefore may be lost. A key example of this would be the failure to prioritize educational activities in the light of a target-driven culture, where one view of what professional practice is about (i.e. the rapid throughput of patients) blinkers its proponents to any other view, and (we would argue) is threatening the quality of both education and health-care. Alternatively, we may sometimes have to concede that our espoused values are unable to be achieved in the current situation, that the case to prioritize them has not been made, that we need to find a compromise position or that they are truly inappropriate. (But we do not think that this is true of the above example – even in the short term.) (See de Cossart and Fish, 2005, Chapter 2)
- Clarified values:
  - are chosen from alternatives that have been carefully considered
  - are consistent with each other (have an internal logic)
  - are limited in number
  - are genuinely able to be put into practice
  - should enhance professionalism
  - should be communicable
  - should be written down
  - need to be revisited, critiqued and developed as understanding grows.

SOME ACTIVITIES TO TRY

To begin to unearth your own professional values, and prepare to write a statement of them, try the following activities:

(A) Write a reflective account of an incident in your own practice that was particularly influential in your thinking about how you should conduct yourself as a doctor, and then list what the incident suggests are important ideas/beliefs/motivations for a doctor to aspire to

(B) Choose someone whose medical practice has particularly influenced how you think about your professional responsibilities and shaped how you wish to conduct yourself as a doctor, and write a descriptive account of what you would wish your practice to emulate

(C) Make notes under the following headings:
- I believe the following are the most important characteristics of a medical practitioner: ...
- I believe that doctors as a matter of principle should aim to: ...
- I think doctors should strive for the following important qualities: ...
- I think that doctors should be people who: ...

(D) Try drafting a first statement of your professional philosophy – about what medical practice should be about and the kind of doctor you will therefore seek to be. (Remember this is something you will need to keep updated as you progress in your career.)

Try these activities in a small group where you each write on your own, but then share each others' writing – NOT to criticize it but to use it to help you extend your own thinking. Also, use the later resources in this chapter to revise and refine what you have written

---

Once doctors have used this resource to tease out further their professionalism in respect of a given case or cases, they might consider comparing their attempt with those of four practitioners in Chapter 4 of Fish and Coles (2005).

A further useful exercise that is worth engaging in from time to time at various career stages is to sit down with the heuristic and Resource 5.1 and to make notes in response to the questions:

- What kind of a doctor do I want to be?   (espoused professionalism)
- What kind am I now?   (professionalism in action)

Having worked on this for a period, a useful activity would be to begin to try to write a statement of one's professional philosophy. The following resource will then help to extend these ideas by raising them to a more general level.

RESOURCE 5.2: BEING A MEMBER OF A PROFESSION

The word 'profession' is still the only precise term for characterizing specialist groups who earn a particular kind of living in an exchange economy. Being a *member of a profession* is far more than merely behaving professionally (which is often used to imply that people are efficient, punctual or well presented). Far

---

Resource 5.2   Membership of a profession (with acknowledgement to Freidson, 1994)[a]

- A profession is an occupation. It is specialized work by which a living is gained
- But it is more than an occupation – it is work for some good in society (education, health, justice)
- A member of a profession exercises a 'good' in the service of another, and engages in specific activities that are appropriate to the aims of the service
- The service that a member of a profession renders a client cannot entirely be measured by the remuneration given
- Members of a profession have a theoretical basis to their practice and draw upon a researched body of knowledge
- Work by a member of a profession is esoteric, complex, discretionary, requiring theoretical knowledge, skill and professional judgement that ordinary people do not possess, may not wholly comprehend and cannot readily evaluate
- Professionals have an ethical basis to their work. This is about much more than having a code of conduct to follow. It is about having to make on-the-spot judgements and engage in actions that are immediate responses to complex human events, as they are experienced. (That is, professionals create meaning on the spot in response to a complex situation.)
- This brings with it the moral duty for the professional to be aware of the values (personal and professional) that drive his/her judgements and actions and the duty to recognize and take account of them as part of their on-the-spot responses
- Being aware of one's personal and professional values is therefore vital
- It also brings with it the need for some autonomy of action. This needs to be circumscribed by the traditions within which professionals are licensed to practise
- The capacity to perform this service depends upon retaining a fiduciary relationship with clients. ('Fiduciary' means that it is necessary for the client to put some trust in the judgement of the professional and the professional needs to inspire such trust.)
- In the public interest, professionals also need to have a commitment to life-long education. This raises important questions about the nature of professional knowledge and about how to enable someone to learn professional practice

[a]Adapted from Fish and Coles (2005).

---

beyond this, membership of a profession commits an individual to subscribe to those general values that are found across all professions.

Membership of a profession: why it is important and what it means

Members of a profession work in practical human settings in which they offer a valuable 'good', or well-being, to individuals and society that is of such value that money cannot serve as its sole measure. Their preparation for their livelihood, their motivation to join their profession and their continuing professional development separate them from other groups who earn a living. Thus, even in the 21st century, their work is different in kind as well as in degree from that of other occupations. It is complex, and so, in the public interest, practitioners need to be educated and assessed by members of their profession in order to enter that profession. To continue within it, they must now be prepared to engage in lifelong development.

Professional practitioners identify closely with their work, such that they develop intellectual interests in it. The work of a member of a profession takes place in practical settings that require the use of esoteric, theoretical knowledge; a researched base; and high-level skill (none of which a lay person can entirely obtain, totally comprehend or fully evaluate). It involves working with people who are vulnerable, and thus demands the professional practitioner's acknowledgement of moral and ethical considerations.

The human situations in which professionals work involve some unpredictability, and so not every element of the work of a professional can be predetermined. Because every person for whom professionals work is particular and individual, professionals must use their judgement. Thus the work of a professional is discretionary in nature. This in turn requires that practitioners have self-knowledge and be aware of their own personal and professional values and the values of their profession.

'Confidentiality', 'etiquette' and 'collegiality' are important concepts in the work of a professional practitioner. Their work requires practitioners to operate within the bounds and traditions of the profession through which they are licensed to practice. Such traditions have been developed over a long period in response to the demands and values of society. Professional bodies are the guardians of these standards, and as such are regulatory.

As we said in de Cossart and Fish (2005), we believe the current demands upon professionals to achieve performance targets are leading to the erosion of these traditional ways of working and being. We would argue that the current demotivation of senior members of professions is probably related to this. Young professionals, those considering such a career and those involved in their education need to give careful thought to this changing world and its effect on the development of the professional practitioner of the future.

Many professions have already recognized that they will fail the public if they allow these crucial characteristics to be obscured and undervalued. Where this is the case, they have built consideration of such matters into their curriculum at all levels.

RESOURCE 5.3: TWO MODELS OF PROFESSIONAL PRACTICE AND THEIR VALUES

This resource raises the question about whether a professional is merely a technician or whether there is more to professional practice than that – and, if so, what it is.

Since models are dangerous because they are reductionist – their chief use is in stimulating discussion. The following polemical model presents two pictures of professional practice in order to explore the views and the values that underlie them. Readers should critique the following, and consider their own position in respect of it. Is there a middle way that is cohesive in its arguments and characterized by as clear a logic as the following? Or must the espousal of some elements of one lead to a rejection of the other? Our view is that technical skills are necessary but not sufficient as the basis for professional practice.

We can see from this resource that professional practice is conceived by some people as involving a set of clear-cut routines and behaviours (performances) and a pre-packaged content that requires merely an efficient means of delivery. Such people argue – value the idea – that this cuts down considerably on the risk that professionals might fail to provide a reliable service. In turn, this makes assumptions that practice is a relatively simple interaction in which the practitioner knows what should happen despite appearing to negotiate with patients or clients. However, this view is seen by others as denying the real character of both professionalism on the one hand and practice on the other. Such people value, and therefore argue for the importance of, complex decision-making and elements of professional judgement and practical wisdom guided by moral principles. They see these as central to the daily work of professional practitioners.

The first view of professionalism is known as the 'Technical Rational' (TR) view (Schön, 1987a). It characterizes professional activities as essentially simple, describable and able to be broken down into their component parts (skills or competencies) and finally mastered. It sees professionals as being essentially efficient in skills, which they harness in order to carry out other people's decisions. This view makes practitioners accountable only for the competencies used within their defined area of practice. However, this means that they are answerable only for the technical accuracy of their work, within the bounds of achieving other people's goals. Thus, in the TR view, the professional's role becomes purely instrumental, and some would argue that this reduces the work of a professional to a sub-professional level, where the right 'behaviour' is laid down for all and is all that matters.

The second view, the Professional Artistry (PA) view (Schön, 1987a), defines professionalism as being concerned with both means and ends. It is concerned to critique the appropriateness of the profession's and the professionals' intentions, as well as the means by which they achieve them. Here, professional activity is more akin to artistry, and practitioners are broadly autonomous, making their own decisions and essentially exercising their professional judgement about both their actions and the moral bases of those actions. In this model, the professional is not

Resource 5.3   Two models of professional practice and their values[a]

The Technical Rational view	The Professional Artistry view
• Follows rules, laws, routines and prescriptions	• Starts where rules fade, sees patterns and frameworks
• Uses diagnosis and analysis	• Uses interpretation/ appreciation
• Wants efficient systems	• Wants creativity and room to be wrong
• Sees knowledge as graspable, permanent	• Sees knowledge as temporary, dynamic and problematic
• Sees theory as applied to practice	• Sees that theory also emerges from practice
• Visible performance is central	• There is more to professional practice than the surface features
• Setting out and testing for basic competencies is vital	• There is more to it than the sum of its parts
• Technical expertise is all	• Professional judgement counts
• Sees professional activities as masterable	• Sees mystery at the heart of professional activities
• Emphasizes the known	• Embraces uncertainty
• Standards must be fixed; they are measurable and must be controlled	• That which is most easily fixed and measurable is also often trivial – professionals should be trusted
• Emphasizes assessment, appraisal, inspection and accreditation	• Emphasizes investigation, reflection and deliberation
• Change must be managed from outside	• Professionals can develop from inside
• Quality is really about the quantity of that which is easily measurable	• Quality comes from deepening insight into one's own values, priorities and actions
• Technical accountability is what matters	• Professional answerability is at least as important
• This requires training	• This requires education
• Takes the instrumental view	• Sees education as intrinsically worthwhile

[a]Adapted from Fish and Twinn (1997).

less but more accountable. Here, to be professional is to be morally accountable for all one's conduct – not just the delivery of the service. Conduct, then, rather than performance, becomes of central value.

It will by now be clear that each view of professional expertise brings with it a different view of (set of values about) what professionals should do in order to learn and then to continue to develop their practice.

The following might be argued, then:

- The TR approach sees skills as central, as relatively simple to learn, as unproblematic to 'apply' to practice and therefore as able to be set down for the professional in protocols.
- It leads to an obsessive intention to tie things down further and further in the inevitably vain attempt to try to cater for all eventualities.
- It argues for the mastery of skills and uses the erroneous claim that skills are 'generic' (implying that they 'transfer'), in order to justify teaching them as if they can be unproblematically utilized in all contexts.
- It values only 'Formal Theory' produced by researchers who, ironically, stand apart from the practitioners whose work they try to shape, such formal theory being learnt and then applied to practice.
- It sees practice as the arena in which to demonstrate previously worked-out theory.
- It uses the language of 'quality control', places emphasis upon visible performance, and seeks to test and measure these, valuing technical expertise as all-important.
- It holds to the idea that learning cashes out immediately into visible products.

Thus the model is behaviourist, and emphasizes fixed standards, and ways of controlling these.

By contrast:

- The PA view values the idea that professional practice is complex, problematic and more than skills-based, and that 'good practice' is context-specific and promotes the idea that treating practice as measurable is nonsense, because what is most easily measurable is often also the most trivial.
- It seeks to develop a professional who has been educated roundly, is not drilled in skills but knows how, when and where to use these skills, and recognizes that skills will always need to be adapted to each new context.
- It recognizes the theory that is implicit in (underlies) all action.
- It sees both action and theory as developed in practice, and that refining practice involves unearthing the theories on which it is founded, while formal theory aids the development of practice by challenging and extending the practitioner's understandings.
- It holds that reflection is the key means of learning to 'do' and of enabling theory to emerge from practice, thus generating an important form of knowledge.

- It treats practice as holistic and complex, and thus values looking carefully at one's actions and theories as one works, challenging them with ideas from other perspectives, and seeking to improve and refine both practice and its underlying theory.
- It encourages the notion that professional practitioners are eternal seekers rather than 'knowers'.
- It believes that there is more to practice than its surface and visible features and that there is more to the whole than the sum of the parts.
- It gives professional judgement a central role in practice.
- It values investigation, reflection and deliberation as a means to enable professionals to develop their own insights, and holds that this is a better means of staff development than innovation imposed from outside (seeing quality as coming from deepening insight into one's own values, priorities and actions).
- It regards the activities of the professional as mainly open capacities that cannot be 'mastered', that involve creativity on the spot, and that thus inevitably involve risk, there being no creativity without risk.

In the PA view then, the professional is working towards increased competence. Such competence is of course grounded in skills – but not to the exclusion of wider capabilities – and is guided by principles, which (unlike skills) are truly generic, being flexible tenets, not rigid rules.

Readers should consider these polar views of professionalism carefully, and then critique them in the light of their own practice as well as critiquing their practice in the light of them.

RESOURCE 5.4: THE VALUES OF A WHOLE PROFESSION

Every profession works on the basis of profession-wide values, whether tacit or declared. The values of any profession emerge over time and have in common the following facts:

- They have historical roots.
- They grow out of an understanding of what is involved in being a particular kind of professional practitioner.
- They are influenced by the developing traditions of professional practice.
- They recognize the values of the current context within which that practice is taking place.

The General Medical Council's (GMC's) *Good Medical Practice* makes explicit the standards, and thus the profession-wide values, for medical practice. It requires all doctors to value the good standards of practice that it describes. It is therefore an important resource for exploring medical professionalism. It is updated regularly, and doctors consulting it should be sure that they have the latest version. It is a response to the concerns of the public and government about the quality of the medical profession, and the prevailing concerns in society about the accountability of members of professions more generally. The RCP's recent report: *Doctors in Society, Medical Professionalism in a Changing World,* also offers some ideas that readers are encouraged to explore. We offer a flavour of these documents in Resource 5.4.

Resource 5.4 The values of a profession

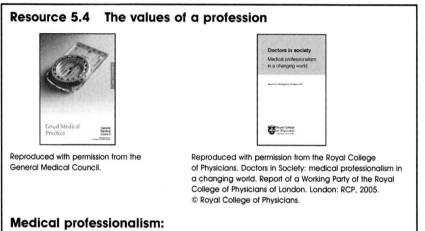

Reproduced with permission from the General Medical Council.

Reproduced with permission from the Royal College of Physicians. Doctors in Society: medical professionalism in a changing world. Report of a Working Party of the Royal College of Physicians of London. London: RCP, 2005. © Royal College of Physicians.

Medical professionalism:

- defines good clinical care and its processes
- makes explicit expectations about clinical judgement and patients' rights to be treated even if they pose a risk to the doctor
- establishes the need to maintain good medical practice and performance
- sets standards of objectivity and honesty and requires sound evidence in the assessment of doctors
- expects all who teach to be able to demonstrate evidence of being a competent teacher
- sets out the conditions for good relationships with patients (consent, trust, confidentiality, communication, ending relationships)
- provides procedures for dealing with the poor conduct or performance of colleagues
- clarifies the expectations for working well with colleagues (treating them fairly)
- recognizes the importance of working well in teams, leading teams, arranging cover, taking up appointments, sharing information with colleagues, delegation and referral
- shapes the minimum requirements for probity (honest information, not pressurizing patients, writing reliable reports)
- requires the protection of patients' care and safety as a first priority in any research conducted.

(See GMC, 2006)

The summary of the RCP report states:

'... The practice of medicine is distinguished by the need for judgement in the face of uncertainty. Doctors take responsibility for these

---

judgements and their consequences. A doctor's up-to-date knowledge and skills provide the explicit scientific and often tacit experiential basis for such judgements. But because so much of medicine's unpredictability calls for wisdom as well as technical ability, doctors are vulnerable to the charge that their decisions are neither transparent nor accountable. In an age where deference is dead and league tables are the norm, doctors must be clearer about what they do and why they do it.

We define medical professionalism as a set of values, behaviours and relationships that underpin the trust the public has in doctors ...'

(RCP, 2005)

The clarification, written statement and regular updating of a profession's values is vital in a number of ways:

- It provides the public and professional regulators with explicit parameters of professional conduct, which can be currently expected of members of that profession.
- It provides educators of new entrants to the profession with the basis for helping them to recognize and scrutinize critically the values of the profession they are joining.
- It provides intending entrants to the profession with a basis from which to consider their own values and the relationship of these to those of the profession.
- It provides teachers, learners, assessors, evaluators and the profession with one starting point for the rationale for professional education.
- It provides curriculum developers with a proper basis for ensuring that all the key elements of the curriculum fully support the values of the profession and the consequent needs of learners.
- It provides examiners and assessors with the basis for deciding the purposes of assessment, what should be assessed and how.
- It provides all relevant parties with a properly explicit basis for review, critique and development of the curriculum itself.

Readers should now consider their statement of their professional philosophy in the light of Resource 5.4.

END-NOTE

The Friday meeting between the Consultant and the SpR

SpR: Hi ... have we got enough time to do this now or are you too busy?

Cons: Yes of course, come in ... sit down ... we'll have about half an hour or so ... I've asked Pat [secretary] to keep things away from my door! Have you got the paper work and your thoughts?

SpR: OK ... well ... yes ... well here is my writing on my professional values in general ... I've brought the heuristic and Resource 5.1 as well ... um, it was not easy to do this and I am not really sure I have given you what you want ... I have made bullet points. I was really not sure how to do this.

Cons: Don't worry this is a starting point ... it is not a test ... just a way in to looking with you at this important aspect of our professional life. Now let's see what you have written ... mmm ... good.

OK, but before we start that let's go back to Mrs Smith and Heuristic 2.

[A conversation then ensues for 15 minutes or so about the SpR's impression of herself with respect to this case and the kind of professional she sees herself as. It is then followed by:]

Cons: Good, OK so there is something there to be thinking about as we go through each of your bullet points.

[They continue in discussion. Examples of a range of typical 'values' the SpR might come up with are in **bold type**. The kinds of challenges and questions the consultant might respond with are in *italics*. Note that the body of the conversation is not included here, because of space constraints.]

- **I am committed to being as good a doctor as possible**
What does this really mean? From whose perspective do you want to be a good doctor? Your own or the patient's? In the interaction on Tuesday, do you think the patient went away with the idea that you were too busy to attend to her specifically? Whose agenda was most important to you at that moment? How does all of this fit into how others see your professionalism?

- **Patient care is my top priority**
I have no doubt that you espouse this, but how do the patient and indeed the other members of staff that you are working with see you doing this? Can you talk again about how the patient and the others with you saw your values on that day? Were they patient-centred or not? How did the juniors see you?

- **I want to do what is good for my career progression**
What do you understand as important for your career progression? Is there a gap between career progression requirements and what you do on a day-by-day basis? Are there ever any conflicts? Do you think my ideas on what is good for your career progression differ from yours?

- **I value honesty and integrity**
I agree, and you do demonstrate that in many ways. That is integrity and

honesty in the public arena. What about integrity and honesty in medical life? It is said that we cover up our mistakes. What do you think?

- **I value the opinion of my seniors about my performance**
What does this really say about how you do things when I am there and when I am not there? Do you change your behaviour for different scenarios related to when I am observing and when I am not?

- **I value the opinion of my peers about my performance**
Do you share your reflections on your cases you have managed with your peers in a rigorous and scholarly way or just in the pub?

- **I value being efficient and getting through the work**
How does that equate to bullet point two.... And how doesn't it?

- **I value being able to teach juniors**
What do you think you taught the juniors about being a busy doctor? Do you think they might have gone away with the idea that efficiency overrides sensitive communication with the patient?

Cons: OK ... well that has been very useful. I am really impressed that you have been prepared and able to engage in a serious and properly critical exploration of your practice and yourself both orally and in writing. Can you sum up what you will take away from this discussion?

SpR: Well ... that it's all rather more sophisticated than I thought, and that I need to think further about the internal logic of my own views ... And that I need to be careful not to undermine the values that matter to me by doing or saying something off the cuff ... I think it's something about *living* one's values ... Oh, and writing these things down has helped us to have an agenda for discussion. It's been good that discussion can wander around many aspects sometimes quite different from what you had first thought about. I had expected a hard time but it has been useful and I will use the ideas to reflect on my own. It has given a lot of food for thought, not least a new language! Thanks for your time.

Cons: Yes. I have found it very useful too; we are all still learning. You might like to take this on by looking at this too. [Hands over Resource 5.3] What you need to do now, perhaps is to explore what others think. I am sure we will come back to this ... but for now back to the patients! See you later.

Commentary

The scene here is well set to encourage an honest, highly motivated and brave discussion from which the learner will gain much. The words used by the consultant at all stages set the scene for a shared and cooperative learning session and establish an atmosphere in which the learner has no hesitation in opening up her difficulties, hesitations and anxieties. The teacher is clearly hoping that what once seemed a simple matter is recognized as complex and worthy of investigation and continued consideration. Thus, this is seen as a sequence of educational sessions.

Having motivated the learner to be actively involved and to commit her ideas to paper so that they can be properly considered and worked upon, the teacher can now adopt strategies designed to help the learner think more carefully, to extend her ideas, to test out their implications and to check out the internal logic of her personal views. However, in working to encourage the learner, the teacher must also be careful not to appear to condone low-level aspirations and ideas unworthy of a maturing professional.

Teachers are themselves models of professional values, in the sense that their activities and the values that underlie them are visible to all with whom they engage in educational and clinical matters. They cannot but offer themselves as an example of 'how to be' in clinical settings and as teachers. Observers will naturally compare and contrast the teacher's values with their own and with the various values statements of the wider healthcare communities of which they are all a part.

So perhaps the teacher has not drawn enough on her own example and experiences of value conflict both within her own practice and across teams she leads, in order to make this a more reciprocal and balanced exploration. Teachers (who will also be clinical supervisors and therefore leaders of the team), should remember that observers only see the smooth running of the surface of their expert practice, and that they need to ensure that the learning doctor understands the processes and thinking that allow their practice to appear effortless. The teacher should therefore value the opportunity to deliberate with the learner about how they have achieved this and encourage the learner to understand how they might fine-tune their own response to the conflicting demands that they will meet in their own clinical practice.

We hope that this scenario, together with the rest of the chapter, has revealed the potential in clinical practice for unpacking without confrontation the professionalism of both educator and learner. We believe that bringing the heuristic and these resources up to clinical practice offers a more profound opportunity for educational development than has hitherto been recognized.

FURTHER READING

Davies C (1998) Care and the transformation of professionalism. In Knijn T, Sevenhuijsen S, eds. *Care, Citizenship and Social Cohesion.* Utrecht: Netherlands School of Social and Economic Policy Research.

Saks M (1998) Professionalism and health care. In: Taylor S, Field D, eds. *Sociological Perspectives on Health, Illness and Health Care.* Oxford: Blackwell Science.

[These two publications show healthcare professionals exploring their professionalism. Both are available, in abridged form, in Davies G, Findlay L, Bullman A, eds. (2000) *Changing Practice in Health and Social Care*. London: Open University/Sage: pp. 343–54.]

de Cossart L, Fish D (2005) *Cultivating a Thinking Surgeon: New Perspectives on Clinical Teaching, Learning and Assessment*. Shrewsbury: tfm Publications: Chapter 2. [This offers an overview, for surgeons particularly, of many of these ideas.]

Fish D, Coles C, eds. (1998) *Developing Professional Judgement in Health Care: Learning through the Critical Appreciation of Practice*. Oxford: Butterworth Heinemann. [This shows a number of professionals across healthcare exploring their professionalism and its significance.]

Fish D, Coles C (2005) *Medical Education: Developing a Curriculum for Practice*. Maidenhead: Open University Press/McGraw-Hill: Chapter 4. [This provides examples of doctors and a nurse teasing their professional values out of individual patient cases they have been involved in.]

Freidson E (1994) *Professionalism Reborn: Theory, Prophecy and Policy*. Oxford: Polity Press.

Freidson E (2001) *Professionalism: the Third Way*. Oxford: Polity Press.

[These latter two books show us how to nurture and develop professionalism in the current climate.]

Southern G, Braithwaite J (1998) The End of Professionalism? *Soc Sci Med* **46**: 23–8. (abridged in: Davies C, Findlay L, Bullman A, eds (2000) *Changing Practice in Health and Social Care*. London: Open University/Sage: 300–7).

Pereira Grey D (2002) Deprofessionalising doctors? *BMJ*, **324**: 627–8.

[Both of these are pessimistic about professionalism.]

O'Neill O (2002) *A Question of Trust (The 2002 Reith Lectures)*. Cambridge: Cambridge University Press. [O'Neill argues the importance of preserving trust between patients and professionals, and the danger of eroding professionalism in the current attitudes of the media and the public.]

6

Understanding the forms of knowledge the doctor uses: Prompted by Heuristic 3

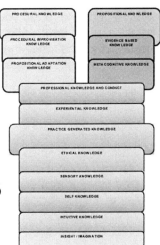

OPENING SCENARIO

You are invited to read this chapter with the following scenario in mind:

> **Consultant (Cons) talking to new Specialist Registrar (SpR) in the outpatient department**
>
> **Cons:** Today we are in the 'difficult leg' clinic, where, as you know, we have many patients whom we care for jointly with the dermatology and haematology departments. That's why it can be very confusing when you start in this clinic. So to help you and to provide a basis for our working together further, I'd like you to do two things.
>
> Firstly, before we start the clinic, I suggest you take a few minutes to write down what you think you need to learn in order to see patients on your own and to plan their care. Bullet points will be fine. Keep the notes you make.
>
> Secondly, after the clinic, I'd like you to write a detailed prose account of one case from this clinic. Then, using this prompt sheet of different forms of knowledge [presents Heuristic 3 and Resource 6.1 to SpR], please annotate your writing by indicating the forms of knowledge you needed to call on to care for that patient. Later in the week I think we should go through this together and use it as a basis for planning your learning programme for this attachment. Is that OK?
>
> **SpR:** Well ... um ... Yes ... Thank you ... That sounds really good ... but I have to admit that I'm a bit nervous about the quality of my writing.

Cons: Don't worry ... For the moment, I am more interested in understanding how you see the knowledge you use and how we can ensure that we offer you appropriate learning opportunities. We might explore your written style later if you like! ... Maybe we could meet on Friday after the ward round in my office to have a look together at both pieces of work?

SpR: OK ... Fine ... I'll start that now ...

Some questions to consider as you read this chapter
- What different kinds of knowledge do doctors draw upon in managing a patient case?
- Why does it matter that doctors become aware of the range of *forms* of knowledge they use?
- Where does doctors' knowledge come from (what are the sources of that knowledge)?
- Do doctors draw on and use knowledge differently at different stages in their careers?

INTRODUCTION

This chapter offers some ways of thinking about the knowledge that underpins clinical practice, and demonstrates that there is far more to this than the theoretical knowledge learnt in medical school. The first main section explores some new ways of learning about the knowledge that underpins medical practice, and also opens up the complexity and importance of what is now generally referred to as 'practice knowledge'. The second section then offers Heuristic 3, which is designed to prompt learners as they begin explore these ideas. This is followed by a series of three further resources to support deeper exploration. The final scenario at the end of the chapter provides one model for how both learner and teacher can explore practice knowledge, using the heuristic, in relation to a given case. It does so by picking up the later meeting between SpR and Consultant as referred to in the opening scenario. The further reading provided at the end of the chapter has been drawn from both the literature of medicine and that of the wider healthcare professions.

NEW APPROACHES TO FOSTERING LEARNING; NEW VIEWS OF KNOWLEDGE

New ways of fostering learning: noticing the difference

While working recently with F2 doctors and their individual consultant supervisors on case-based discussion, we taped (with permission) a number of conversations between the pairs as they were filling in the required forms. Many of these, when replayed to both parties and to the wider study group to which they belonged, revealed two excruciatingly obvious problems that needed to be addressed, but which were not even recognized, let alone resolved, during the discussions. These problems stemmed from widely differing assumptions about the purpose of the exercise, and resulted in highly divergent agendas that clearly became a barrier to learning, but that were highly illuminating to the whole study group. The details were as follows.

Each member of the pair brought sharply contrasting mindsets about the spirit in which the case was brought for discussion. Supervisees came as part of a new programme in which they were just beginning to take more responsibility for their learning. They thus appeared with a case *to share* with their teachers in the hope that exploration of it with a more experienced doctor would prove enlightening in respect of real practice. But the supervisors (still trapped in the hard-to-break habits of the older style of more hierarchical medical education) viewed the supervisees as *'reporting'* to them. These differing mindsets (captured in the words 'sharing' and 'reporting'), resulted in noticeably different tones of voice, which made the dialogue uncomfortable for both parties. On the one hand, supervisees had been led by the new curriculum to see education in and for the clinical setting as an enterprise in which teachers and learners would work cooperatively together. But, on the other hand, supervisors saw it as a subordinate reporting to a senior as a means of checking out their actions and as an excuse for teacher to further test learner's 'knowledge' (i.e. their medical theory), some of which was only loosely connected to the case, and also as an opportunity to offer their own superior knowledge.

This dichotomy, of course, is also related to two quite different ideas about what the 'content' or focus of the teaching should be. The supervisees were looking for help in thinking more clearly *about a specific patient*. They saw it as a chance to extend their experience and understanding of real practice. They seemed to want to talk about more than the theory they should bring to the management of the patient case. But the supervisors were using the case as a springboard from which to quiz the supervisees on the adequacy of their medical/clinical/theoretical knowledge *about the generality of such cases*. They saw it as another means of preparing the learning doctors for their exams and a chance to highlight the factual medical knowledge needed to pass them. We believe that this is not untypical and that if this exercise were carried out within specialist training, similar findings would be revealed.

What this highlights in particular is how deeply embedded in medical education is the view that medical factual knowledge (theory) plus the ability to carry out medical processes (practice) are all that matter in exploring a patient case and coming to decisions about its management. But, as we shall show in this chapter, that is far from so. Further, we believe that it is important to challenge this view of medical knowledge as merely 'theory plus practice', because for so long as that limited view of knowledge remains implicit and thus unexamined in the minds of teachers and learners, it will be hard to release postgraduate medical education into more realistic ways of thinking about medical practice and more creative modes of learning.

Developing the Wise Doctor

By contrast to this, the approach taken by the consultant in the scenario at the start of this chapter, and which is pursued further at the end, shows the teacher engaging the learner in some short but specific and achievable activities that are intentionally designed to involve and motivate as well as provide the concrete resources for a well-informed later discussion. Indeed, the design of these activities is particularly powerful. The initial list that the learner was asked to prepare will, when shared later, reveal to both of them the learner's starting points, while the annotated case from the clinic will have helped the learner to come to grips at their own speed with both the new ideas and language for considering them, and will have got them ready for the planned developmental discussion, which can now start at a much higher level.

Further, the learner's writing will provide, for a range of audiences (self, other portfolio readers, patient, general managers, colleagues or risk managers), some irrefutable evidence of learning. By getting the learner to write down both what they already know and think, and then asking for a case to be recorded and annotated in writing, the teacher is establishing sound and lasting evidence of the learner's starting points, learning needs and, ultimately, progress, for them both to see and consider. It also ensures that there are good concrete resources to aid learning through the later discussion.

There is, of course, an expectation on the part of the teacher that there will be a discrepancy between what the learner believes about the kinds of knowledge they will need, and the much broader range that they will discover is actually required in clinical practice. And because of the design of this whole educational endeavour, the learner is doing the work, is becoming engaged in it, is discovering for themself (which is always more persuasive and memorable than 'being told' by someone else), is 'teaching themself' – with some guidance – and is learning how to begin to investigate their practice, which will ultimately enable them to take over their own personal development. Clearly, this is a way of turning *teaching* into *learning* in respect of the knowledge that doctors draw upon in the clinical setting.

However, the learner's ability to grasp all this without the consultant being present all the time is dependant upon having readily available the prompt and the key resources that will aid the learner's exploration of these ideas about knowledge (see Chapter 3). This is the role of heuristic 3 and resource 6.1. It should be noted, however, as we have said before, that this is not an argument for distance learning. Subsequent discussion with the consultant is a vital component to enable understanding to be identified, critiqued and developed. This should be the more enjoyable for both parties because the ground work has been done, the consultant's time, that would have been taken up in presenting these new ideas, has been saved and the learner has been able to work at their own pace through the early stages of coming to grips with new ideas and language.

New views of knowledge: introducing practice knowledge

Knowledge has traditionally been seen as consisting of two simple components: theory (propositional knowledge, or 'knowing that *x* is the case') and practice (procedural knowledge, or 'knowing how to do y'). This twofold division may currently still be the basis of the structure of undergraduate medical courses, but because it is very simplistic, it does not get us very far in developing postgraduate medical practice or other forms of healthcare practice. Indeed, although medicine is only now beginning to realize it, a much wider range of kinds of knowledge lies under the thoughts that doctors have and the interpretations and decisions they generate about patient cases. Indeed, such a plethora of kinds of knowledge is now recognized as underpinning professional practice, that the term 'practice knowledge' is commonly used to refer to the whole field.

Heuristic 3 has been developed because there is more to knowledge than we readily see and more than doctors have in the past discussed as part of a patient case. This is because much of doctors' knowledge is implicit or even tacit. If clinical practice is to be developed (and developed faster than it was in the past), the knowledge that underpins the thinking and the decision-making of doctors needs to be made explicit and further explored in respect of specific patient cases by both teachers and learners.

In patient cases where the condition is common, where there is one obvious way of managing the medical problem, and where the patient is otherwise fit and well so that there are few if any medically confounding factors, the knowledge that fuels doctors' thinking may be mainly procedural and propositional knowledge, and this, together with some reference to evidence-based knowledge, is used by trainees in a standardized and well-rehearsed way. This approach is regarded as the foundation of learning to manage successfully more complex cases.

Cases are rarely that simple, however, and apparent simplicity can, if taken at face value, be the beginning of problems for doctor and patient. Further, more complex cases are likely to require the use of most if not all the knowledge described in heuristic 3. Interestingly, in such complex cases, doctors often draw on only a small amount of propositional and straightforward procedural knowledge and are often astounded in retrospect by the range of other kinds of knowledge they have used. Thus, it cannot be too soon for the new doctor to begin to explore the more complex elements of practice knowledge.

INTRODUCING HEURISTIC 3

Why do practitioners need heuristic 3?

We would argue that there are five main reasons why practitioners need a working understanding of practice knowledge. This can be gained by using heuristic 3 to explore practice. They need to:

- identify, explore and understand the knowledge that drives their decisions and actions
- have readily available the language and the concepts endemic to exploring knowledge for the purposes of teaching, learning and assessment

- explain the basis of their recommendations to patients (whose own *medical* knowledge has expanded exponentially as a result of the Internet, but who do not have either the depth of understanding, or the wide range of other knowledge that characterizes a wise medical practitioner)
- discuss the knowledge that underpins their practice with colleagues and members of the wider healthcare community
- develop their practice, expand their awareness of their moral and ethical approach to practice, and promote a critical examination of that practice.

They need a working understanding of practice knowledge because: 'the practice setting is a vital arena for the construction of new knowledge by practitioners themselves' (Higgs *et al.*, 2007). They also need to be articulate about these matters because the nature of knowledge drawn upon and generated within the practice setting is complex in the following ways (de Cossart and Fish, 2005, p. 186):

- It is always incomplete.
- It is characterized by mystery at its heart (some of it being tacit).
- It evolves during the collaborative relationship with colleagues and clients and often within practice itself.
- It involves theorizing about practice *during* practice.
- It is about creating new understandings *during* practice.

Heuristic 3: content and design

Practice knowledge is now understood to contain some subdivisions of theory (e.g. evidence-based knowledge), and some subdivisions of practice (e.g. knowing how to improvise within procedures and how to adapt medical factual knowledge to non-standard cases). But it also includes some forms of knowledge that cannot so readily be described as 'entirely theory' or 'entirely practice' but that are very important. Examples of these include experiential knowledge, knowledge of professional regulation and traditional conduct, knowledge generated as a result of being in the practice setting (not only audit and research, but also smaller but significant new personal insights about either 'facts' or 'ways of doing something'), ethical and moral knowledge (both how to reason properly within this field of knowledge and what to factor into such reasoning), knowledge gained through the senses of touch/smell/sight/sound, self-knowledge, intuitive knowledge, and knowledge gained from 'putting oneself into another's shoes' (insight/imagination). Those who doubt the significance of intuitive knowledge are referred to Claxton (2000).

Heuristic 3 is designed to set out these forms of knowledge as if on a pack of cards, in a logical and memorable way in order to prompt the learner to remember and identify them in respect of a patient case that has been selected for deeper exploration. This heuristic needs to be used together with the resources that follow it, particularly Resource 6.1, which expands these ideas in more detail by offering a map of knowledge that doctors use.

On examining Heuristic 3, readers may be surprised by several aspects of its design. For example, we have started at the top with two columns where we have deliberately separated procedural knowledge (practice, or 'knowledge of how to do *y*') which is placed in the left-hand column, from propositional knowledge (theory, or 'knowledge that *x* is the case'), which appears in the right-hand column. Thus readers meet 'practice' cards before 'theory' cards. We have done so in order to challenge the traditional order of the phrase 'theory and practice', which implies that theory always comes first for a learner. We have done so because we believe that often it is practice that actually comes first for learners and in the creation of new knowledge, and that we carry out some activities (e.g. riding a bike) quite without the theoretical knowledge that underpins our performance (e.g. prior knowledge of the laws of balance).

This idea is traditionally referred to in the phrase 'the primacy of practice'. It is Gilbert Ryle who called our attention to the arguments for the primacy of practice. In his seminal book, *The Concept of Mind*, he challenged the traditional relationship by declaring: 'Efficient practice precedes the theory of it … It is … possible for people intelligently to perform some sorts of operations when they are not yet able to consider any propositions enjoining how they should be performed.' He added: 'Some intelligent performances are not controlled by any interior acknowledgments of the principles applied to them (Ryle, 1949, p. 31). Further he said: 'we learn *how* by practice, schooled indeed by criticism and example, but often quite unaided by any lessons in the theory' (Ryle, 1949, p. 41).

He is not, of course, saying that there is no knowledge underlying such actions, but rather that the knowing is *in* the doing, that is, that the (factual) knowledge used is often unknown or lies beneath our consciousness, and is a part of the action rather than separable from it. This must mean that some factual knowledge is learnt in and during practice, not before it. And it is why the theoretically proposed division between theory and practice cannot be sustained in 'real life'.

Forms of knowledge that combine theory and practice are particularly important for learning doctors, but are usually tacit. It is why we have placed these kinds in the lower part of our heuristic. It is also why in that single column of cards, the 'practice-generated knowledge' card appears deliberately larger than all the others.

The use of heuristic 3

We recommend that both learners and teachers use heuristic three to remind them to explore a case that has been deliberately selected because it will repay a depth of study. We suggest that the knowledge cards be used to help identify the range of forms of knowledge used in treating and managing the patient, and that the case be used to challenge the content of the knowledge cards and to illuminate and critique practice (thus employing theory to critique practice, and vice versa).

It should be noted that not all cases draw upon the entire gamut of these kinds of knowledge and also that a relatively small number of cases, explored in depth by learners in terms of the knowledge base that the doctor is using, will enable learners to become familiar with these ideas and use them within clinical practice.

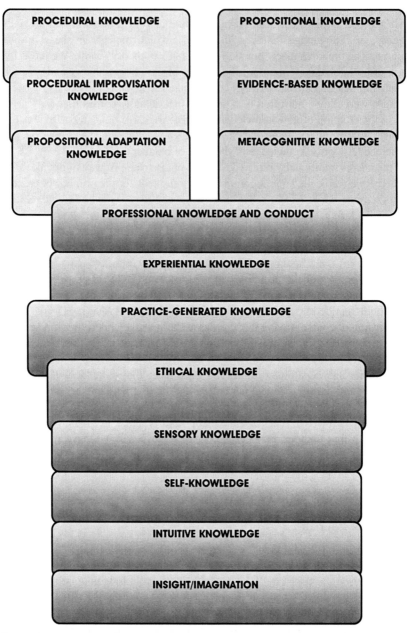

Figure 6.1 Heuristic 3: the knowledge cards (Fish and Coles, 2005, p. 142). Affected and shaped by values, and always context-specific to the clinical setting.

THREE RESOURCES TO PROMOTE EXPLORATION OF THE HEURISTIC

Resource 6.1: A map of practice knowledge for doctors

Resource 6.1 has been placed next to Heuristic 3 because it offers more detail in respect of each form of knowing and is designed to enable the finer detail of the

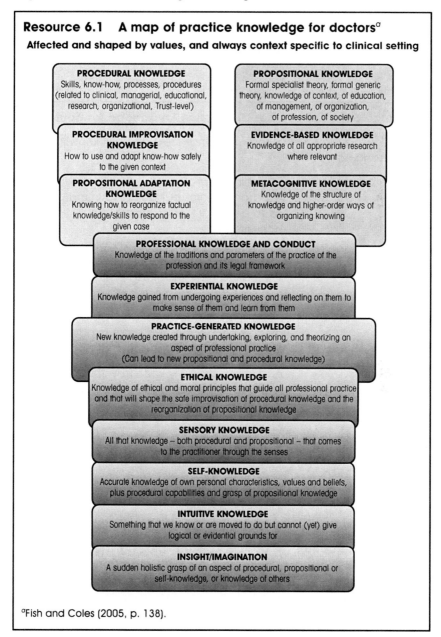

Resource 6.1   A map of practice knowledge for doctors[a]

Affected and shaped by values, and always context specific to clinical setting

PROCEDURAL KNOWLEDGE
Skills, know-how, processes, procedures (related to clinical, managerial, educational, research, organizational, Trust-level)

PROPOSITIONAL KNOWLEDGE
Formal specialist theory, formal generic theory, knowledge of context, of education, of management, of organization, of profession, of society

PROCEDURAL IMPROVISATION KNOWLEDGE
How to use and adapt know-how safely to the given context

EVIDENCE-BASED KNOWLEDGE
Knowledge of all appropriate research where relevant

PROPOSITIONAL ADAPTATION KNOWLEDGE
Knowing how to reorganize factual knowledge/skills to respond to the given case

METACOGNITIVE KNOWLEDGE
Knowledge of the structure of knowledge and higher-order ways of organizing knowing

PROFESSIONAL KNOWLEDGE AND CONDUCT
Knowledge of the traditions and parameters of the practice of the profession and its legal framework

EXPERIENTIAL KNOWLEDGE
Knowledge gained from undergoing experiences and reflecting on them to make sense of them and learn from them

PRACTICE-GENERATED KNOWLEDGE
New knowledge created through undertaking, exploring, and theorizing an aspect of professional practice
(Can lead to new propositional and procedural knowledge)

ETHICAL KNOWLEDGE
Knowledge of ethical and moral principles that guide all professional practice and that will shape the safe improvisation of procedural knowledge and the reorganization of propositional knowledge

SENSORY KNOWLEDGE
All that knowledge – both procedural and propositional – that comes to the practitioner through the senses

SELF-KNOWLEDGE
Accurate knowledge of own personal characteristics, values and beliefs, plus procedural capabilities and grasp of propositional knowledge

INTUITIVE KNOWLEDGE
Something that we know or are moved to do but cannot (yet) give logical or evidential grounds for

INSIGHT/IMAGINATION
A sudden holistic grasp of an aspect of procedural, propositional or self-knowledge, or knowledge of others

[a]Fish and Coles (2005, p. 138).

patient case to be teased out. It can be used as an *aide mémoire* to talk through or to write in more detail about the patient case. Both this resource and the heuristic should be treated with criticality and thus used to explore practice but also to be the subject of critical scrutiny in the light of practice.

Resource 6.2: The sources of practice knowledge for doctors

Resource 6.2 seeks to identify the sources of these different kinds of knowledge. This might be of use where a learner identified an area of weakness in their thinking about practice knowledge and needed to pursue it back to source.

Resource 6.2 The sources of practice knowledge for doctors[a]

The following are sources/resources that feed doctors' knowing and understanding:

Service commitment	Engaging in professional practice in theatre, ward and clinic, but doing so 'mindfully', so as to be aware of at least some of its components: • improvising procedural knowledge • adapting propositional knowledge • creating new knowledge during practice • professionals as models of various kinds
Practising procedures	Repeating procedures and processes, but reflectively, so that this is not mindless repetition of practice irrespective of quality
Reflection	Analysing critically actions, thoughts and knowledge embedded in practice, particularly in relation to own practice and experience
Those outside the service commitment	• Written knowledge: books, journals, research papers, internet • Oral: lectures, talks • Demonstration • Master classes • Dictats (government, national and local)
Personal interaction	• Learner asking probing questions and using talk to clarify understanding • Engaging in professional conversations • Induction into the traditions of practice enshrined in professional conduct of

---

	senior colleagues, by discussion with and observation of them • Discussion with the interprofessional team in theatre, clinic, ward
Self	• Experiential, personal and professional experiences reflected upon • Sensory (observation and tactile, auditory and olfactory senses) • Memories of experiences and patterns • Intuition • Insight
History and narrative	• Anecdotes of earlier cases • Making a narrative of an episode of practice and enriching it with the help of reflection, and of others who were there
Education	• Being taught • Being supervised • Resource-based learning (plus discussion with teacher) • Observing practice • Engaging in practice together with reflection • Using own educational portfolio • Being assessed • Learning to self-assess

[a]de Cossart and Fish (2005, p. 200).

An interesting way to begin using this resource is to ask the learning doctor to consider which sources of knowledge he/she uses during the course of a given week. In order to emphasize the point, the exercise should be set prospectively not retrospectively, and the doctor should be asked to keep a daily record.

Resource 6.3: Some thoughts on how doctors use knowledge differently at different learning stages

Teachers and learners might use the following thoughts (Resource 6.3) to help them explore further some elements of the learner's knowledge-base, not in terms of facts, as is so often the case, but in terms of the sources and nature of knowledge more generally. This also provides a range of references that could be followed up by anyone wishing to gain more information about these matters.

> **Resource 6.3   Some further thoughts about how doctors use knowledge**
>
> Eraut and du Boulay have pointed out that there is evolution of both knowledge structure and diagnostic skill as postgraduate doctors become more experienced. What is more, they imply that in postgraduate medical practice, learning new ways of structuring the knowledge already possessed takes precedence over accruing large amounts of new propositional knowledge.
>
> They state, for example, that increase in postgraduates' *knowledge* of pathophysiology is small compared with the reorganization of that knowledge already known, to make it more readily and rapidly available (Eraut and du Boulay, 2000, 3.1.1).
>
> They acknowledge that the work of Chang *et al.* (1998) had emphasized this previously.
>
> Quoting Grant and Marsden (1988), Eraut and du Boulay also remind us that every practitioner's knowledge base is highly individual and will have evolved from their previous personal clinical experience.
>
> The knowledge of novice doctors is largely scientific in nature, and has been structured for them by its presentation in textbooks and lectures that highlight the intrinsic structure of the academic discipline. Few teachers in medical school invite learners to restructure this for themselves (make it their own). Postgraduates gradually have to find their own way of repackaging their knowledge to enable it to be drawn on quickly and appropriately in their everyday clinical practice.
>
> Schmidt and Boshuinzen (1993) set out a model for considering the difference between novices and experts and their use of knowledge. They say that being an expert is not knowing more than novices but merely organizing knowledge differently, combining it with increasing experience of cases, until the cases become more significant than the scientific knowledge. Medical educators need crucially to know where their learner is with respect to this, in order to help them to develop further.
>
> Saliency is at least as important as erudition. In all this, it should be remembered that 'expertise lies not in the knowledge *per se*, but in the judgement of what's pertinent and important' (Cox, 1999, p. 277).

FINAL SCENARIO

Consider the following both in respect of one way a learner might use heuristic 3 (together with Resource 6.1) and in respect of the model it offers of how this material might be taught. This is, of course, only one possible model, and is not to be copied. Rather, the underlying principles of good teaching should be unearthed from it and used as a guide (see also Chapter 3).

Postscript to Chapter 6: Friday morning

Cons: Ok, let's see what you have come up with. How did you find the whole exercise?

SpR: Well it was more difficult than I thought. But this is what I did.

Firstly here are my bullet points listing what I thought I should learn about:

- Read textbook on leg ulcers
- Read about deep vein thrombosis (DVT) and post-phlebitic limbs
- Review my reading on dermatology
- Read the protocols for leg ulcers and DVT on the hospital Trust intranet
- Talk with you about what you like to be done to your patients.

Cons: I'm not surprised to see what you have written. It is largely about gaining facts about the disease isn't it? Though I'm pleased to see the last one! How does the list compare with what has come out of your writing?

SpR: Ah well, yes there's certainly lots of other kinds of knowledge here. I've tried to highlight them in red, but I'd welcome further help....

The case:

... Mrs S was a 29-year-old woman who had a DVT in her first pregnancy four years ago and has been seen regularly in this clinic because of a swollen leg. She is keen to get pregnant again and wants to come off the warfarin. She is wearing a support stocking. She is a teacher. **[Mainly propositional with some procedural knowledge]**

I read through her notes and learned that she had three miscarriages before her successful pregnancy, but there was no thrombophilia screen in the notes. She has been advised by the consultant in the past that she would be wise to avoid further pregnancies. **[Propositional knowledge]**

Clinical examination **[procedural knowledge and sensory knowledge]** *revealed a fit, slim woman with a swollen left leg and good foot pulses.* **[Propositional and procedural knowledge]**

*I discussed with her the risks of recurrent DVT in further preg-
nancy, which I had checked out in my textbook. Interestingly,
there is little helpful **evidence based information** on what to
do here, but there was a useful protocol for the management
of anticoagulation in pregnancy on the intranet **[propositional
knowledge]**.*

*I sensed on talking to her that she is very upset at having only
one child. It seems that both her husband and she were only
children and did not want their own child to miss out on having
siblings as they had done. **[Insight/imagination/sensory
knowledge]** I was surprised how convincing I found her argument for a further pregnancy .*

*I agreed to talk to you and the haematology team and come
up with a plan for her anticoagulation if she is determined to go
down that route. I think she understood the risks **[ethical knowl-
edge]**. I have seen one patient managed in this way throughout a pregnancy and it was OK **[experiential knowledge]**. I
have referred her to our multidisciplinary meeting **[profes-
sional knowledge]**.*

Cons: Yep. Interesting. That looks about right. You are using the
resources well. So, can you summarize what you learned from doing
this, then perhaps at the end we'll go on to look at why it might
matter to be able to do this and finally at how to shape your learning agenda for this clinic. ...

SpR: Well ... I suppose I have learned that some patients can put
a very convincing argument for their case even though they see the
risks. That was something new and challenging to me.

Cons: And what kind of knowledge is that?

SpR: Er ... well ... I suppose its um ...

Cons: Well, ... how about **practice-generated knowledge**?

SpR: Oh ... I see, ... I wondered what that really meant. Yes ... of
course, I came to it during practice ...

Cons: Good. And what are the moral and ethical aspects that this
case presents to us as doctors? ...

Commentary

The underlying principles here are that the discussion should be cooperative and
positive in tone, that it should seek to acknowledge the learner's achievements
and take the thinking on, that wherever possible it should be the learner who

makes the main points, that the learner should summarize, that silence should be used as a means of encouraging thinking, and that the agenda for learning should emerge between teacher and learner as a result of the learner analysing what they know and what they yet need to learn about.

FURTHER READING

de Cossart L, Fish D (2002) Membership of a profession Part Two: The nature of professional knowledge in medical practice, *Mersey Deanery Newsletter* **14** (2). Liverpool: Mersey Deanery. [This short article offers an example of the identification of practice knowledge in respect of a case of breaking bad news.]

de Cossart L, Fish D (2005) *Cultivating a Thinking Surgeon: New Perspectives on Clinical Teaching, Learning and Assessment.* Shrewsbury: tfm Publications: Chapter 9. [This chapter offers more theoretical detail on the nature of practice knowledge.]

Claxton G (2000) The anatomy of intuition. In: Atkinson P, Claxton G, eds. *The Intuitive Practitioner: On The Advantages of Not Always Knowing What One is Doing.* Maidenhead: Open University Press: Chapter 2. [This chapter explores what is involved in intuition, and does so in very useful detail.]

Fish D, Coles C (2005) *Medical Education: Developing a Curriculum for Practice.* Maidenhead: Open University Press: Chapter 7. [This chapter offers more detail on the nature of professional knowledge in medicine and its implications for the postgraduate medical curriculum.]

Higgs J, Andressen A, Fish D (2004) 'Practice Knowledge – its nature, sources and contexts. In: Higgs J, Richardson B, Abrandt Dahlgren M, eds. *Developing Practice Knowledge for Health Professionals.* Oxford: Butterworth Heinemann. [This chapter unpacks the nature of practice knowledge for professionals across the whole of health care, and shows that the language and ideas related to practice knowledge as offered in this book are consonant with those available to the multiprofessional team.]

Higgs J, Fish D, Rothwell R (2007) Knowledge generation and clinical reasoning in practice. In: Higgs J, Jones M, Loftus S, Christensen N, eds. *Clinical Reasoning in the Health Professions.* Edinburgh: Elsevier: Chapter 15. [This chapter provides a state-of-the-art overview of healthcare's current understanding of how practitioners generate practice knowledge.]

7

Illustrating the quality of the doctor's clinical thinking: Prompted by Heuristic 4

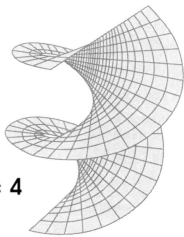

SCENARIO FOR WORKING WITH HEURISTIC 4

This uses the story from Chapter 6.

Cons (to the same SpR):   We have already used the knowledge cards to review the different forms of knowledge that we use everyday in clinical practice, and I think you did well and that we both learned a lot. Now I would like extend this to explore your clinical thinking. Oh, and by the way, your writing's not at all bad!

Taking the case you used for the knowledge cards, since we are both familiar with it now and the patient is due to be discussed at the Multi-Disciplinary Team (MDT) meeting, would you familiarize yourself with the elements of the Clinical Thinking Pathway (Resource 7.1), look at this Resource (Resource 7.2) and then construct your own table in two columns to summarize your own thinking. The heuristic of the helicoid is a reminder of the complexity you are going to begin to unpack.

Your table should look like this: the left-hand column should contain the elements of the Clinical Thinking Pathway ... the right-hand column should be reserved for the clinical aspects of the particular case you are exploring.

The elements of the clinical thinking pathway	The key aspects of my thinking in this case

Now, I think I've framed *the complex clinical problem* correctly as follows:

A 29-year-old woman, on warfarin because of a previous DVT, which has left her with a very swollen left leg. She has one child and is desperate to have a second. You have made the decision to refer her to the MDT meeting to consider her wishes.

… So you'll be able to start there …

Perhaps we could go through this together on Tuesday before the MDT meeting.

SpR: OK. Great … Thanks …

Some questions to consider as you read this chapter

- What is involved in arriving at sound decisions about the management of patient cases?
- How can I make explicit, critique and develop the thinking that leads up to the key decisions I make in the clinical setting?
- Why is it important to do this?
- What is the difference between a clinical decision and a professional judgement?

INTRODUCTION

Clinical thinking does not simply lie at the very core of any professional's practice. It *is* the core of it. But it is invisible, being hidden from all observers. Doctors are responsible for making the most major and far-reaching clinical decisions and professional judgements about patient management. Their ability to come to sound decisions and to explain and defend them is central to success. These decisions take account of highly complex, unpredictable and problematic details, as well as exercising specialist thought processes drawn from the sciences and the humanities. This involves far more than is (or can be) taught at medical school. Postgraduate doctors need access to how clinical thinking works in practice. But often instead, they are provided by their seniors with only the end-results of such thinking – with the clinical and professional conclusions reached in respect of each specific patient. How they discover and make sense of what has led up to these, and how they can learn to make such decisions themselves, often seems to be left to chance.

We are arguing that learning how to surface, explain, explore and refine the detail of the thinking behind medical decisions – especially complex ones – is central to postgraduate medical education and that it requires special support both from teachers and from resources that have been tailored to this need. Such resources must offer both the ideas and the language through which clinical thinking can be developed.

This chapter attempts to provide both those ideas and that language. It does so by explaining why clinical thinking is important; by arguing why it involves far more than is learnt at undergraduate level; by offering a framework for exploring it and a language in which to discuss it; and by providing (both in the opening and closing scenarios as well as within the main sections of the chapter) ideas of how it might be taught.

For example, the scenario at the start of this chapter shows the teacher able to save the valuable teaching time, usually devoted to telling the learner the basic facts, by sending the SpR off with some key resources and a task specifically designed to enable her to become really familiar with the complexities of clinical thinking. Using knowledge, rather than just receiving it as handed down from the teacher, is a key to genuine learning.

In respect of the strategies adopted in this scenario, we note how, in order to support the solo learner, the teacher carefully prepares the groundwork for doing the task. She makes very clear how to set out the table required; offers a detailed example of how to start it; and sets a time for this exercise to be discussed between them. In thinking about this case, the teacher has ensured a sequence of educational development for the learner in both content and activity. The development of the content ranges from using the knowledge cards in respect of a case to investigating the clinical thinking involved in the same case. The development of activity sees the teacher *inviting* the learner to engage in working solo, and then sharing the ideas so that they can be challenged and extended. By these simple means, the learner is provided both with a sense of continuity that is so often missing in learning in the clinical setting, and with a strong sense that the work she will do will be acknowledged and valued. And the teacher's invitation is far from a coercion, in that it offers the promise of learning together and motivates the learner to prepare for this.

THE IMPORTANCE OF ARTICULATING CLINICAL THINKING

Few would reject the statement that: 'Arriving at sound professional decisions in complex clinical situations is a key and unavoidable responsibility of the professional, and the exercise of such duty usually separates professionals from laymen' (de Cossart and Fish, 2005, p. 132). Clearly, learning doctors must acquire this ability as a priority. But the problem is that the end destination (reaching 'sound professional decisions') often obscures the importance and complexity of the processes of 'arriving at' those decisions.

The significance of sound professional decisions, then, is paramount. Doctors are accountable for their actions, and the decisions and reasoning that led to them in respect of patient care. Most importantly, they have both a duty and a responsibility to maximize these abilities in order to care properly for patients. In addition, they need to be able to identify the sound decisions of colleagues, both peers and juniors. Further, given the litigious nature of our society in the 21st century, doctors' decision-making processes are also often the starting point for prosecution and defence in cases where medical error is being investigated. For all these reasons, doctors need to be clear-thinking and articulate about any key decision they make (see also RCP, 2005).

Disentangling *how* a decision was arrived at (and therefore being able to defend it robustly), however, is not so easy. For doctors particularly, the contextual information, the patient narrative, the professional knowledge and the scientific evidence that fuel their thinking are all inevitably incomplete and/or require interpretation and sensitive reprocessing, and then have to be further customized to the individual patient and the individual patient's case, because all practice is context specific. As Sackett *et al.* (1997, p. 4) argue, there can be no 'cook-book' solutions here, because medicine:

> 'requires a bottom-up approach that integrates the best external evidence with individual clinical expertise and patient choice, it cannot [therefore] result in slavish cook-book approaches to individual patient care. External evidence can inform, but never replace, individual clinical expertise and it is this expertise that decides whether external evidence applies to the individual patient at all, and if so, how it should be integrated into a clinical decision.'

We would argue that, by contrast to experienced doctors, inexperienced ones are often characterized by remarkable, but unfounded, *certainty* about clinical matters, and lack awareness of both the frequency of the need for good professional judgement and the complexity of the reasoning that leads to it. Once in practice, they need as soon as possible to seek to recognize and confront the complexity of situations by learning these reasoning processes.

But this is not easy. Until now, learners have mostly been left to grasp the principles of sound clinical thinking and good judgement exercised silently and invisibly by their seniors, and to try to develop their own facility in them, by osmosis. For example, consultants, as clinical supervisors, often announce the results of their own clinical decisions, leaving learners to observe their visible actions, but without making them privy to the *whole* of the thinking that underlies decision and action, or perhaps no longer being conscious of the detail of it. Or such teachers make explicit or ask the learner to give a commentary about *only* those elements of reasoning that are overt, or that can easily be articulated and described most straightforwardly. At worst, this can unintentionally mislead learning doctors about what is really involved in the vital processes of clinical thinking, and at best it does not do justice to the complexities of real medical practice.

It is also the case that, until recently, assessments of the learning doctor's clinical reasoning, deliberative processes and professional judgement have only been carried out implicitly within more general assessments of the learner's work in clinical settings. It has neither drawn on hard evidence of nor generated any detailed records of achievement in this area. This state of affairs has not promoted enduring confidence from the wider audience. Neither does it match the growth of understanding of such matters (including assessment of them) in many of the other professions allied to medicine. And it will certainly not be sustainable in the face of increased governmental surveillance of medicine in the 21st century. It therefore seems clear that these are crucial processes, which doctors now need to be taught directly and assessed in rigorously. As we have said in relation to surgical education (de Cossart and Fish, 2005, p. 134):

> 'All this sets a particular challenge for the medical educator who must be able to surface, and make explicit and discuss the details of these hitherto tacit and taken-for-granted processes, who must find ways of enabling learners to understand and exercise them, and who then must encourage open ways of capturing and assessing them, so that achievement in them can be recorded and understood by new teachers and colleagues later in the young ... [doctor's] career.'

CLINICAL THINKING: INTRODUCING HEURISTIC 4 – THE HELICOID

This heuristic (the helicoid – Figure 7.1), which indicates the complexity of a pathway associated with a helix, is designed to prompt readers to consider the whole process of 'arriving at' the key decision(s) they wish to explain, explore and/or defend. The point here is that there are many pathways up and down the two surfaces of the helix, and this reminds us that different routes can be taken in either direction. This is important, because when we set out a simple version of

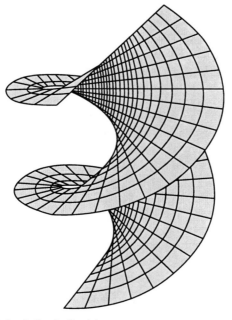

Figure 7.1 Heuristic 4: the helicoid.

the Clinical Thinking Pathway in order to explain its elements, we do so in a linear fashion, for clarity's sake. Inexperienced doctors will initially need to learn to discuss the elements of their thinking by following this linear pathway, but when experienced doctors engage in the process, they move up and down the pathway freely, as appropriate to the complexity of the case.

The elements of the Clinical Thinking Pathway follow, as the first resource. These arise from our explorations, in the clinical setting, of the key components of clinical thinking, and their basic relationship, as found in practising doctors. We are not suggesting that these processes themselves are in any sense new, but rather that we have clarified the elements involved, which hitherto have been mainly tacit, and offered a language in which to discuss them, and how they come together holistically in the expert practitioner. This, we believe provides a foundation from which inexperienced doctors can explore their thinking and that of their seniors and thus develop and refine their abilities to articulate the arguments behind their major professional decisions.

It should be noted that, throughout this chapter, we use the phrase 'clinical thinking' to encompass the entire process of the doctor's thinking, from meeting the patient to making a professional judgement about their management.

An overview of the pathway (Resource 7.1)

This pathway falls into two main sections. In the first part of the pathway (starting from the top) the thinking processes, which we refer to as 'clinical reasoning', are scientific. They lead up to a clinical solution. This overall process provides a framing of the problem, collecting and interpreting the available evidence, coming to a diagnosis, and reaching the *general* solutions for this problem as found in the medical textbook. Simple versions of this thinking are taught to undergraduates in medical school, but its complexities are only really available to postgraduate doctors. The second (bottom) half of the Clinical Thinking Pathway, which we refer to as 'deliberation', is based upon humanistic thinking and enables the doctor to engage in weighing competing priorities in order to tailor the general information provided via the scientific thinking, to the patient's specific needs. This whole thinking process can really only be learnt by a postgraduate doctor who is already taking real responsibility for patients.

As we shall see, these two ways of thinking are greatly contrasting in nature.

Clinical reasoning

In its simplest and purest form, *clinical reasoning* construes the complex clinical problem as a *technical* one. It then operates through a formula designed to solve purely clinical problems and thus comes to a *clinical conclusion* by using a straightforward set of rules. The assumption here is that what counts as evidence in the given case would be agreed by everyone.

Clinical reasoning can be seen as a biomedical process that distinguishes the disease from the patient and regards the problem as to do with malfunctioning

Resource 7.1   The elements of the Clinical Thinking Pathway[a]

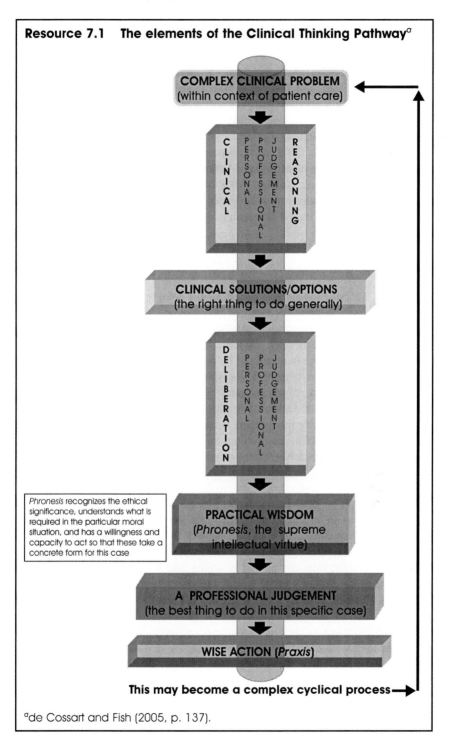

COMPLEX CLINICAL PROBLEM
(within context of patient care)

CLINICAL PERSONAL PROFESSIONAL JUDGEMENT REASONING

CLINICAL SOLUTIONS/OPTIONS
(the right thing to do generally)

DELIBERATION PERSONAL PROFESSIONAL JUDGEMENT

Phronesis recognizes the ethical significance, understands what is required in the particular moral situation, and has a willingness and capacity to act so that these take a concrete form for this case

PRACTICAL WISDOM
(*Phronesis*, the supreme intellectual virtue)

A PROFESSIONAL JUDGEMENT
(the best thing to do in this specific case)

WISE ACTION (*Praxis*)

This may become a complex cyclical process

[a]de Cossart and Fish (2005, p. 137).

parts of the patient. It is a technical problem, requiring *technical* competence from the practitioner. It is based on logic and order, collects predictable categories of evidence, and uses a formulaic approach to reach a clinical decision. It claims a scientific basis, and stems from a worldview that sees facts as objective, precise and absolute, and 'Truth' as 'out there', waiting to be discovered. It assumes that scientific theory can be directly translated into practice. And it is deliberately devoid of moral and ethical concern.

But when 'the simplicities of science come up against the complexities of individual lives' (Gawande, 2001, p. 8), personal professional judgement has to be exercised and other important forms of clinical reasoning in response to a complex clinical problem are needed. For example, even in the most technical of patient cases, investigations must be selected; evidence must be interpreted and explanations found for it; and judgements must be made about when enough evidence is at hand.

Deliberation

By contrast, *deliberation* always recognizes the complexity at the core of clinical thinking, and sees clinical problems as humane problems, which are inevitably characterized by messiness and uncertainty, and which require an echoing human response from the practitioner. Deliberation holds as an open question what would count as evidence in respect of its arguments. Doctors at the start of their career who have not recognized deliberation as a significant process of clinical thinking during medical school are often shocked to discover its central importance in medical practice. Deliberative processes include: recognizing all the relevant elements; accepting the humane nature of the problem; contextualizing it; seeing multiple views of it; interpreting; prioritizing and attributing significance. The final product of this deliberative process is the professional judgement that is made together with colleagues and patient. We focus on this in more detail in Chapter 8.

A key example of deliberation is the process that turns a working diagnosis into a treatment plan for a particular patient. Deliberation, then, is grounded in the professional's humanity and is concerned with the patient's social being in the world. It calls upon imagination and compassion in the practitioner to help him/her understand how the patient is seeing and feeling. It sees disease as a breakdown of the patient's social world, and crucially recognizes that the meaning of any situation is likely to be construed differently by each of the different people involved in it.

Deliberation draws on the artistry of the practitioner. That is, it involves recognizing the unique nature of the situation, engaging in a dialogue with that situation, and being ready to go beyond the rules (Schön, 1987a, p. 22). It is based on pragmatic and practical reasoning in which human and equally competing priorities vie for attention, in an order *that has to arise from the particulars of the problem* and that will therefore be different for different patients. It thus eschews formulae for thinking, using instead an investigative approach to unearthing all the pertinent elements and a reflective and critical approach to prioritizing and weighing them up.

In summary, then, the following can be said:

1. Clinical reasoning is biomedically based and rational. It includes: knowing what counts as evidence; requiring technical competence; using positivistic logic; assuming a stable world; seeing order as important; adhering to formulae; regarding facts as objective and absolute and truth as 'out there waiting to be discovered'; applying theory to practice; and excluding moral and ethical issues.

2. Deliberation is humanities-based and interpretative. It involves: starting from practice and the patient; seeing the world as subjective and uncertain; negotiating what counts as evidence; requiring artistry; using practical reasoning; prioritizing pragmatically; attending to sharply competing demands; admitting multiple versions of reality and knowledge as socially built; interpreting significance; and accepting responsibility for focusing on moral and ethical issues.

The main components of clinical thinking

We see the process of clinical thinking as beginning with the identification of the *patient's complex clinical problem*. This should be distinguished from a relatively uncomplex medical issue and its resolution. In such a simple problem, what is arrived at would be a 'medical decision'. This would be a response to answers to closed questions about fairly uncomplicated activities or issues. A medical decision might be: 'Shall I put up a drip here? Shall I order a CT scan? Shall I prescribe drug X or Y?' (de Cossart and Fish, 2005, p. 135). Equally, a personal/career decision might be about whether or not to apply for a given job, or might require the choice between attending an educational seminar on which one was booked or an extra ward round that has occurred opportunistically. Here, only fairly simple pros and cons need to be considered before a clear-cut decision, which is quickly self-validating, is made. There is no weighing of considerable numbers of equally competing complex priorities.

Senior doctors make medical decisions tacitly and fast. Learners may need to rehearse the pros and cons aloud and check out their appropriateness and that of the decision reached, but this can be done quite thoroughly through brief discussion at the time. A 'medical decision' is not, therefore an element of the Clinical Thinking Pathway.

The complex clinical problem and its formulation

A complex clinical problem is the trigger for clinical thinking. It may be a problem that is directly related to the patient, or it may be about an aspect of hospital Trust policy that indirectly affects the patient. It is construed by the doctor, alone or in consultation with patients and colleagues, as the start of the clinical thinking process. Such 'case formulation' draws upon the doctor's (patient's and colleagues') values, beliefs and experience.

Although they are presented in simple terms in Resource 7.1, none of the thinking processes endemic to clinical reasoning and deliberation is actually simple. Indeed, there is a need in each of them, at all points, to identify the salient features involved, to weigh the significance of various elements, and to interpret the meaning of even the most scientific of evidence. This even includes the formulation of the complex clinical problem itself. It involves adjudicating between conflicting priorities, where soundness of common sense and steadiness of focus are essential. Further, all human situations are constantly evolving, and there is always a need for professionals to continue to respond to developments and to refine or reconsider their conclusions. Thus the doctor's vital capacity to exercise *personal professional judgement* is a response to complexity, competing demands, and the ambiguities that all too often arise in evolving human interaction.

A caveat

We believe that these key elements and their basic relationship as mapped in Resource 7.1 are the foundation of any kind of clinical thinking that begins with the formulation of a complex problem and ends with the start of, or plan for, wise action (although of course some elements will be present in greater or lesser degrees depending on the nature of the problem). Thus, this general pathway can be used to explore such thinking, whether it is focused on the process that leads from the first outpatient consultation to an agreed treatment plan; is concerned with the thinking that leads to wise action *within* the treatment itself; or is looking for the resolution of wider clinical issues.

We wish to make it clear, however, that this model (like all diagrams) simplifies and reduces real-life complexities. (This is the point of heuristic 4.) We have presented the pathways in linear fashion, but would strongly emphasize the fact that in real practice, clinicians will always revisit the decisions and the thinking that led to them, when elements that do not fit emerge. This will be especially so when the diagnosis at the end of the clinical reasoning pathway is still somewhat uncertain. The first decision being made at this point enables the progression of care of the patient, but is not necessarily the final diagnosis. (This of course adds to the difficulties that learning doctors have in tracing these thought patterns.) We wish also to make clear that we do not see these processes as solitary activities leading to decisions by lone professionals.

However, we believe we have provided a starting point for thinking about, and a language for discussing, what has until now been only partially attended to.

USING RESOURCE 7.1

Learning doctors may wish to use this resource to help them to understand the whole, or elements of, their thinking processes. They or their teachers might turn it upside down and start with the professional judgement learners have made, and then use the pathway to investigate how they came to that judgement. During the early stages of becoming familiar with this resource we recommend a considerable amount of oral discussion, combined with and based upon brief notes. But the logic and detail in clinical thinking is considerable, and cannot be remembered in enough detail in an oral discussion alone. Because of this, we cannot stress enough that attempts at writing a full account of their thinking in respect of a number of patient cases will repay the learner far more fully. This is because there will always be more to discover through and as a result of the actual process of writing. Many examples of the use of this resource can be found in de Cossart and Fish (2005, Chapters 7 and 8). The following two resources will also help to enrich doctors' exploration of their clinical thinking.

RESOURCE 7.2: AN EXAMPLE OF HOW TO MAP THE PATHWAY OF CLINICAL THINKING IN A NEW OUTPATIENT CONSULTATION

Resource 7.2 is designed to support oral discussion with a supervisor or as a mode of self-assessment, to check out whether all of the necessary clinical thinking processes have been attended to in relation to a given case.

In de Cossart and Fish (2005), we offered three diagrams of the main components of clinical thinking in relation to three different scenarios: the new outpatient consultation; during treatment as a result of a new complex problem arising; and the wider issues of clinical practice (management/systems problems that arise in relation to a specific patient case). We offer here the first of these, for the outpatient consultation, fully annotated with the general details (principles) of what needs to be attended to in coming to a major judgement about treatment.

Learning doctors and their clinical supervisors may like to take this pattern and annotate it instead with the details relating to a specific case. This is an example of another way of recording and thus being able to explore in detail these complex matters. It can combine bullet points with a diagram to flesh out the key details. Supervisors can see quickly from this the quality of the learning doctor's thinking and also pinpoint any element that has been omitted.

RESOURCE 7.3: ADVICE ON HOW TO GO ABOUT EXPLORING YOUR THINKING IN WRITTEN NARRATIVE

Resource 7.3 offers advice that we first provided for surgeons in de Cossart and Fish (2005), but that is equally appropriate for doctors more generally. It is designed to show the order in which to go about unravelling the information, and indicates the level of detail needed in order to construct a narrative that illustrates the doctor's clinical thinking in relation to a particular case. Clearly, the advice is offered in chronological order.

A written narrative is the most useful way of exploring clinical thinking in respect of a complex case. Further, such writing will repay additional thought and

Resource 7.2   The clinical thinking involved in an outpatient consultation[a]

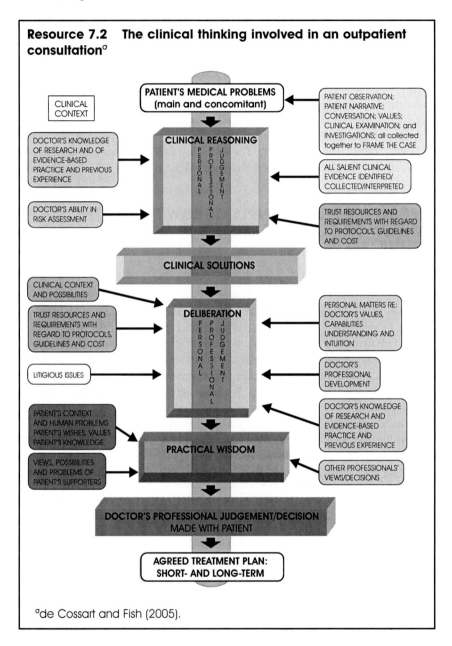

CLINICAL CONTEXT

PATIENT'S MEDICAL PROBLEMS (main and concomitant)

PATIENT OBSERVATION; PATIENT NARRATIVE; CONVERSATION; VALUES; CLINICAL EXAMINATION; and INVESTIGATIONS; all collected together to FRAME THE CASE

DOCTOR'S KNOWLEDGE OF RESEARCH AND OF EVIDENCE-BASED PRACTICE AND PREVIOUS EXPERIENCE

CLINICAL REASONING
PERSONAL PROFESSIONAL JUDGEMENT

ALL SALIENT CLINICAL EVIDENCE IDENTIFIED/ COLLECTED/INTERPRETED

DOCTOR'S ABILITY IN RISK ASSESSMENT

TRUST RESOURCES AND REQUIREMENTS WITH REGARD TO PROTOCOLS, GUIDELINES AND COST

CLINICAL SOLUTIONS

CLINICAL CONTEXT AND POSSIBILITIES

TRUST RESOURCES AND REQUIREMENTS WITH REGARD TO PROTOCOLS, GUIDELINES AND COST

DELIBERATION
PERSONAL PROFESSIONAL JUDGEMENT

PERSONAL MATTERS RE: DOCTOR'S VALUES, CAPABILITIES UNDERSTANDING AND INTUITION

LITIGIOUS ISSUES

DOCTOR'S PROFESSIONAL DEVELOPMENT

PATIENT'S CONTEXT AND HUMAN PROBLEMS PATIENT'S WISHES, VALUES PATIENT'S KNOWLEDGE

DOCTOR'S KNOWLEDGE OF RESEARCH AND EVIDENCE-BASED PRACTICE AND PREVIOUS EXPERIENCE

PRACTICAL WISDOM

VIEWS, POSSIBILITIES AND PROBLEMS OF PATIENT'S SUPPORTERS

OTHER PROFESSIONALS' VIEWS/DECISIONS

DOCTOR'S PROFESSIONAL JUDGEMENT/DECISION MADE WITH PATIENT

AGREED TREATMENT PLAN: SHORT- AND LONG-TERM

[a]de Cossart and Fish (2005).

redrafting. For this reason, it should be noted that following through the list provided in Resource 7.3, in relation to a given case, is not a once for all activity. Both the cases themselves and the writing about them need to be worked over.

Resource 7.3   Constructing a clinical thinking narrative

Constructing a written narrative to demonstrate understanding and critique of clinical thinking

- Seek to construct the story just as it is remembered (doing so as soon as possible after it has happened)
- Start with the facts (these are fairly easily told orally)
- Write them down in the correct order as far as memory allows
- Map them onto the pathway (Resource 7.1)
- Get help and prompting about the facts from others who were present
- Add in brackets, behind each fact captured, the detail of the thinking that underlay your actions (do this in another colour or font and number the points)
- Look at the thinking processes you have surfaced so far, and enrich the facts you have captured, so as to make your *actions* more explicit
- Go backwards and forwards between the facts about your actions and the thinking that you recognize beneath their surface, using each to critique and expand the other
- Work over these and keep refining and adding the details as you remember them
- Keep working over the chronological order (our memories don't work in strict chronological order)
- Be sure you have you distinguished between various kinds of thinking and have offered a critique of the processes you engaged in
- Write the critique at the end of your narrative, using the numbered points to identify the elements you are discussing.

The importance of revisiting decisions and thinking at all stages

We have presented the pathways in linear form, but would strongly emphasize the fact that in real practice, clinicians will always revisit the decisions and the thinking that led to them, particularly when elements do not seem to fit. This is why the helicoid is a useful heuristic. Such movement up and down the Clinical Thinking Pathway will be especially important when the decision at the end is still somewhat uncertain. The first decision being made at this point enables the progression of care of the patient, but is not necessarily the final diagnosis. Indeed, where at any stage uncertainty remains about the accuracy of diagnosis or final judgement, recycling through the pathway must always be carried out. We give an illustrative scenario of this in de Cossart and Fish (2005, Chapter 7).

END-NOTE

The SpR and Consultant meet for discussion of the task set in the opening scenario.

SpR: ... This has been another challenging exercise. It took me a few goes before I got into the swing, but then I got the hang of it. I hope that it is what you expected. I have added shading to distinguish between the clinical reasoning and the deliberation, and since it was my first attempt I have put the various elements of the thinking pathway in the left-hand column and fitted in the elements of the case in the right-hand one. Perhaps I could take you through it.

[SpR shares a copy of the paper with the consultant.]

Cons: ... yes please do. It looks as though you have been very thorough.

The elements of clinical thinking	Key aspects of the clinical case
(Reasoning in light grey, deliberation in dark grey)	
Framing the case From patient narrative, clinical examination, observation and investigation (Part of reasoning – but already 'given')	*This is a 29-year-old woman, on warfarin because of a previous DVT, which has left her with a very swollen left leg. She has one child and is desperate to have a second. We have made the decision to refer her to the MDT meeting to consider her wishes.*
All salient clinical evidence identified/collected/interpreted	General fitness of patient otherwise OK
Risk-assessment exercise	Risk of further thromboembolic complications with new pregnancy; need to weigh up all points in this
Review of literature and other evidence	Fit and well woman with young child. Synthesis of research all emphasizes the risk to mother and new baby of the pregnancy

The elements of clinical thinking	Key aspects of the clinical case
Trust resources	Expertise within the Trust to manage her through such a pregnancy is no problem
Doctor's previous experience	Only one previous case. Need senior help
Doctor's ability in risk assessment	Need to look up literature

CLINICAL SOLUTION: Despite currently well patient, the general advice here would be to avoid further pregnancies in order not to incur further thromboembolic complications or even death.

Patient's context, wishes, values, knowledge	Clear cut end points PREGNANCY or NOT. Patient focused on a new pregnancy
Patient's supporters: Human aspects of the case; values and wishes of her husband	Complex! Husband wants new baby but not to be left as a single parent. Opinions of the rest of the family divided
Further professional involvement/decisions	The gynaecologist's opinion significant – needs to agree
Further professional involvement/decisions	The haematologist's opinion significant – needs to be supportive
Further professional involvement/decisions	GP and midwife need to be supportive
Litigious issues	Clear recording of understanding of woman about the risks of this venture must be undertaken
Doctor's values/capabilities, understanding and intuition	Must consider own values with respect to patient and the problem. Why did patient ask the doctor for advice?

PROFESSIONAL JUDGEMENT/DECISION: many discussions to be had before making decision about whether she should get pregnant. (THIS is a judgement in itself.)

> **Cons:** ... did this exercise bring up any points that you had not thought about in the clinic? Perhaps more particularly, are you clear about what you want out of the MDT tomorrow? ...

Comment

As with all these scenarios, it is only possible to give an impression of the teaching and learning possibilities that can arise from the educational task that has been set. Here the possibilities are considerable. (See Chapter 3.)

FURTHER READING

de Cossart L, Fish D (2005) *Cultivating a thinking surgeon: New perspectives on clinical teaching, learning and assessment.* Shrewsbury: tfm Publications: Chapter 7. [This chapter offers many illustrations of how this pathway can be used, and many examples of how it can be used to present a case in writing.]

Montgomery K (2006) *How Doctors Think: Clinical Judgement and the Practice of Medicine.* Oxford: Oxford University Press: Chapters 4–6. [These important chapters explore clinical judgement and the idea of cause.]

8

Demonstrating the quality of the doctor's professional judgements: Prompted by Heuristic 5

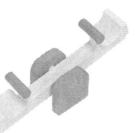

OPENING SCENARIO

You are invited to read this chapter with the following scenario in mind:

> The starting point of this learning opportunity is a complex surgical case that was managed on the day the following discussion took place and that had involved the consultant, John (an F2 doctor), Jane (an SpR Year 1) and Michael (an SpR Year 5). The patient was 45 years old and had presented with peritonitis secondary to diverticulitis and a perforated colon. He had been resuscitated and then taken to theatre, where he had undergone a laparotomy, colonic resection and colostomy. He was now on the High-Dependency Unit.
>
> The scene is the next morning, after the ward round. (This whole scene takes less than 12 minutes.)
>
> **Cons:** So ... the patient from last night seems to be doing well. Good. ... Now, ... I would like us to use this opportunity to focus particularly on the kinds of professional judgements we made in relation to this case, and to think about the quality of those judgements.
>
> I know you have all already explored your clinical thinking processes in relation to other cases, ... and I believe that you now know the basic difference between a relatively simple clinical decision and a key professional judgement; (Yes? Fine) and I hope you are all comfortable now with the two different kinds of professional judgement ... personal professional judgement (which is in process throughout our thinking); ... and the final product of that thinking, which is a professional judgement that will lead to wise action. (Yes? ... good) ...

So tomorrow I'd like us to share and explore together the range of professional judgements we were each responsible for making in this case ... ummmmm ... Let's have a look briefly at this chart ... [offers Resource 8.3] ... As you'll see, it provides a way of considering the *quality* of professional judgements (both the processes and the product).

[*A brief discussion of the chart takes place to confirm that everyone has understood it, and to enable all learners to use the basic language that has been referred to by the consultant, and that they are all comfortable with it.*]

OK ... so ... in preparation, I would like each of you tonight to take about 20 minutes to think about this chart in relation to one aspect of your care of this patient, which I am going to highlight for you ... John, you examined the patient at my instigation and with me watching you yesterday. Be ready to tell me about what judgements you made with respect to how you went about examining the patient. (It was a process professional judgement, wasn't it?) ... Jane, you organized the tests for this patient, so can you describe the professional judgements you made in relation to ordering these tests. ... Michael, you operated on Mr Murray. Would you write about the judgements you made about the operation you were going to perform ... and anything that changed those decisions.

In the education session tomorrow, we'll discuss decision-making and professional judgement, and your contribution will be to share your specific examples and any critique of them, with us ... so that we can think together about them ... and we might also critique the chart I have given you ... OK? ... So see you tomorrow. If you are still not sure what to do, I will be available in my office this afternoon.

Some questions to consider as you read this chapter
- What characterizes quality professional judgements?
- How can I learn to pinpoint my key judgements?
- What exactly are personal professional judgements and how can I explore them?
- How can I 'unpack' the final professional judgements I make, and develop them?

INTRODUCTION

Professional judgement is about achieving a fine balance in the difficult circumstances of a given case. It involves: weighing up complex priorities; discarding some elements; prioritizing others; and coming to rest at a judicious decision that can be well defended and that most people would agree is the best balance possible, given all that must be considered in the given case. Thus, it is about 'practical reasoning' (the kind of reasoning that responds to the pragmatic) and which can only be learnt in practice and through concrete examples drawn from practice. In the past, it was learnt through the accretion of experience gained across hundreds of cases while working beside a senior whose own judgements were recognized as wise, and whose ways of thinking gradually permeated the learner's mind. Today, there is little time for learning all this, and if anything, the judgements to be made are even more complex.

This chapter aims to support doctors in exploring their own judgements and thus improving their awareness of the process and refining the quality of their decision-making, all of which will conduce to better clinical practice and enhanced patient care. We seek to do this by offering an exploration of what is involved in professional judgement for doctors, by setting out some ideas about how this might be taught (by reference to the scenario at the start of the chapter) and by offering a heuristic followed by three learning resources. The chapter closes with a scenario that is a follow-up to the opening one and by offering some further reading.

WHAT IS INVOLVED IN PROFESSIONAL JUDGEMENT FOR DOCTORS?

The Clinical Thinking Pathway distinguishes between two sorts of professional judgement that are made by doctors: personal professional judgement, which is a process in use throughout the whole of the thinking pathway; and a professional judgement, which is the end-product of the thinking and which represents an arrival at a choice of actions that are calculated to lead to wise practice. The following is both a reminder and an extension of the detail offered in Chapter 7.

Personal professional judgement (a process)

Personal professional judgement runs throughout the pathway in which, in respect of a given case, the doctor first seeks to formulate the patient's clinical problem and finally comes to a wise resolution about the best action possible.

This 'process' judgement harnesses a range of kinds of thinking, including common sense and the understanding gained through experience, in order to construe the case in hand as a humane as well as a technical problem. For example, during clinical reasoning, personal professional judgement might cause the doctor to recognize and take account of the fact that there is no one absolute way of interpreting particular evidence, that the patient's story is only one way of making meaning out of a situation of complex meanings that are culturally determined, or that some elements of a case history need to be revisited. During the deliberation process, professional judgement will be called on at all the moments when adjudication has to take place between competing priorities, when ambiguities have to be resolved, or when relative significance has to be assigned to several competing arguments.

A professional judgement (a product that leads to wise action)

The final professional judgement is a decision about the best action to be taken in this particular patient's case. It is the end result of the whole process of clinical thinking. As we have already pointed out, it combines the answers to the questions: What *ought* to be done *in this case*? What *can* be done *in this case*? and How shall we go about doing it *in this case*? And it leads into *wise action or practice*.

Such a judgement may be reached either with the direct input of the patient or be fed into a more conclusive discussion with the patient, which results in an agreed treatment plan (a final decision about the way forward for this individual patient in the light of his/her context and individuality). Equally, a professional judgement may be a decision about a course of action during the treatment, or it may be the final judgement about how best in a given hospital Trust to go about altering a given policy.

HOW WE CAN EXPLORE PROFESSIONAL JUDGEMENT?

Some general points

Clinical supervisors and all other medical/surgical teachers should remember that their overall educational aim is to develop young doctors as independent sources of judgement within their own role in the practical setting. Such doctors need to become self-critical, independent learners, who are also willing and able to engage in clinical thinking, not only to resolve immediate clinical problems in respect of a given patient, but also even to respond to wider professional issues in the service of patients, at the level of public debate and policy-making. Clinical supervisors should therefore choose teaching strategies and resources that do not undermine these aims. This means not feeding learners with facts because it is the quickest and easiest thing to do, but rather engaging them actively in exploration of their decisions.

To develop good decision-making generally, learners should be prepared to become active, rather than passive receivers of information. They should bear in mind the following guidance, which we have adapted from Kirk and Cox (2004, p. 146) (see de Cossart and Fish, 2005, p. 153). Learners should:

- prioritize tasks, regularly reconsider their order, focus on the decision in hand and always be willing to favour the real emergency
- view the problem from a distance, look for inconsistencies, and seek evidence that disproves the decision one is inclined to or habitually favour
- welcome rather than reject uncertainty and recognize the inevitability of complexity (even, suspect that which seems simple)
- not lightly ignore or leave to one side those elements that do not fit one's developing decision
- think carefully about the relative significance of elements
- look at the patient (and the Clinical Thinking Pathway) as a whole
- not rush to identify resemblances between this case and previous ones.

Demonstrating the quality of the doctor's professional judgements

Since practical reasoning is the basis of professional judgement, it should be practised by both teachers and learners. Practical reasoning is built up through extending, elaborating and refining the criteria by which actions are to be justified, and showing how these criteria are to be weighed in practical situations. A tradition of practical reasoning (sound professional judgement) will grow and be available for learners to access once professionals have written down, collated and discussed examples of practice, once gifted individuals have offered insights into their own thinking and when new possibilities have been discovered by experimentation. That is why sharing examples is so important, and why there can be no textbook approach to this.

There are, however, some useful teaching strategies that can help both teachers and learners. These can be identified by studying examples of successful teaching. The opening scenario offers a number of these.

The importance, in the opening scenario, of the teaching and learning strategies

Having spotted a good learning opportunity, the teacher in this scenario has set up a two-stage educational session with great skill. She has given the whole enterprise a clear direction, leaving no doubt about her intentions by making an explicit statement of her aims, and by doing this at the very start. These aims are clearly educational in respect of both the content to be learnt and the activities that the learners will engage in. The content (focus) is on the quality of the learners' professional judgements within a given case. The processes in which she will engage learners are highly educational in ensuring their active involvement in preparing and thinking out their own contribution – which they will do separately – and then using these to teach each other in a shared and sheltered learning environment (clinical practicum) (de Cossart and Fish, 2005, p. 53). She is thus making a virtue of having to teach at the same time three doctors who are at three different stages of experience, she is saving herself from doing all the work, and is at the same time giving them ownership of the session.

The context for learning is well provided by the teacher who, by reminding learners about the work they have all already done at a variety of appropriate levels about their clinical thinking, establishes that this task follows logically from their previous discussions and explorations. She also takes this opportunity to summarize the key language with which the learners should already be familiar.

A new learning resource is then handed out, and the teacher prompts a discussion of it, ensuring that everyone joins in fully. Significantly, this occurs *prior* to setting the task for which the resource will be used. The timing of this allows learners to focus exclusively on the resource, to assure themselves that they have fully understood it and that they are indeed comfortable with the language they have previously learnt. Indeed, the learners' talk enables them to make their own meaning out of what they have been offered, and allows the teacher to check that that meaning-making has resulted in an appropriate result. Talking by learners, rather than by the teacher, is vital at points such as this.

The learners are then ready for the task to be set. The teacher importantly stimulates motivation for learning by indicating that the task will only take 20 minutes that evening, and that by 'sharing' and 'exploring further' their discoveries the next day, they will develop their understanding together in an unthreatening context.

Further, in setting the task, the experience of the learners is carefully taken into account. The task for everyone is to explore the quality of an aspect of their professional judgement in relation to the specific case. All are then offered help in pinpointing a judgement of their own that will repay the time spent exploring it. Here, the teacher has chosen to introduce the complexities of professional judgement by herself helping them out with the most difficult aspect (pinpointing the judgement itself) and by getting them to engage with the easier and more 'fun' elements of exploring a judgement they have made.

This general task of exploring the quality of a professional judgement of their own is then properly *differentiated* across learners in relation to their different career stage and individual ability (see Chapter 3). Here the teacher has appropriately graded the difficulty of the tasks set, to take account of each individual's level, while also maintaining a group approach to the topic. Thus, the F2 doctor is given a simpler task, and, almost as an aside, is gently helped to categorize it ('It was a personal professional judgement, wasn't it?'). By contrast, the more experienced learners were given progressively more demanding examples to explore and were not helped with categorization.

The nature of the task is also interesting. The chart is offered to help critique practice in the interests of improving it, but there is too the suggestion that practice and experience might also be used to critique the chart, in the interest of refining thinking about these matters. Here the teacher is acting as a good model in flagging up the need for criticality and the need to focus such criticality both on their practice, and also on the 'theory' they are offered.

Finally, it should be noted that this whole 'setting-up' process took less than 12 minutes, but that the teacher presented these new ideas at a pace that enabled the learners to take them all in, and gave them a chance to explore them for themselves. She also supported them with paperwork where they could not have been expected to remember the complex details. Her final act of support is to provide a safety net for anyone who is still not clear about the task: '... I'll be available in my office this afternoon.' This teacher is ensuring that the learners' time will not be wasted during their 20 minutes' preparation because they are unsure of the task or the resource.

The resources that the teacher uses, then, in this 'resource-based learning approach', are crucial in enabling her to send the learners away to use their time profitably, to learn better as a result, and to save her doing their work. It should not be forgotten that, using her professional judgement as an educator, she astutely chose as her starting point not the first resource offered below, but the third.

The following pages offer a further range of resources for enabling learners to explore their judgements. These begin with a heuristic to prompt the learner to remember the significance of professional judgement. This is followed by three learning resources: (i) an example of how to learn to pinpoint those final judgements that lead to action, which is an important ability when contacting the consultant in the middle of the night and at handover times; (ii) a table to help recognize the personal professional judgements that colour the doctor's thinking throughout the pathway; and (iii) a table (which the teacher offered learners in the above scenario) that is designed to fuel discussion about, and exploration of, the quality of both kinds of professional judgements. These resources are followed by a short narrative through which we seek to emphasize the need to keep all judgements under review. The completion of the scenario begun at the front of this chapter, together with some further reading, conclude these ideas.

INTRODUCING HEURISTIC 5 (Figure 8.1)

This heuristic (both the picture and the words) are designed to remind the reader that key components of professional judgement are weight and balance. As we shall see below, this becomes crucial in the explorations supported by resources two and three.

RESOURCE 8.1: LINDA'S STORY (TWO VERSIONS) THAT DEMONSTRATES HOW TO PINPOINT JUDGEMENTS

As is clear from everything we have offered in this book, case narrative is a key means to understanding and refining all the elements that lie at the core of medicine, and patterns across cases illustrate and give evidence of the development of

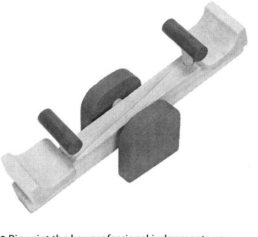

- Pinpoint the key professional judgements you have made in this case and exlore them
- What did you weigh in the balance in coming to your final judgement?

Figure 8.1 Heuristic 5: the seesaw of professional judgement.

insight. In respect of professional judgement, we believe that the pattern across cases will create evidence of someone's whole practice ability.

The following story, offered in two versions, provides an example of a consultant struggling to make explicit the actual key judgements she made in respect of a given case. This particular activity may be as hard for consultants, whose judgements are often implicit, as it is for less experienced doctors. Further, it is an example of a very early piece of reflective writing by the consultant!

Here is the first attempt (Resource 8.1a), in which Linda neither states clearly the key judgements to be made nor offers the detail of how she came to them. This story is typical of what experts will offer about their practice when asked to 'explain it'. Indeed, quite possibly in the working lives of most senior clinicians, their formulation of the initiating complex clinical problem is rarely stated overtly.

Resource 8.1a   Cancelling a patient's operation on the day of surgery (Version one)

It takes more than just knowing about the condition and being able to do the operation.

The case scenario

It was a Tuesday morning at 8 AM, and I arrived to review the patients on my all-day operating list. The previous Friday, I had reviewed the list, and it showed a patient with an abdominal aortic aneurysm from my vascular waiting list and two patients from the common waiting list for thyroid surgery. On the Monday, I had been working away from the Trust. Late on the previous Friday, one of the patients listed for thyroid surgery had phoned to cancel their operation because of a concurrent medical problem. In order not to miss the operating space, a patient requiring recurrent incisional hernia surgery was given the place left by the cancellation. This new patient was admitted to the ward on the Monday and consented by the trainees ready for theatre on the Tuesday. I enquired why another thyroid patient had not been added and was told that this patient was next on the list. I visited the patient for the hernia repair on the ward. His case notes were very thick and were being read very carefully by the consultant anaesthetist. I observed that the patient walked with a stick, and he told me that he was very disabled with joint problems. After a short conversation with him, it seemed to me that both he and I were less informed than we should be about his surgical problem. This was my first knowledge of him. His understanding of the possible postoperative events that might complicate his recovery was very limited. I made the decision to postpone his case and arranged to see him again the following Friday in my outpatient clinic. There was a feeling abroad that I was over-reacting.

Note that this 'outline' story is quite short, and took little more than 10 minutes to write. Note, too, that while the complex clinical problem is not stated in clear and simple terms, it certainly lies implicit beneath the surface. Yet precision of formulation of such key thinking is crucial to shaping the rest of the decisions and actions about treatment.

Resource 8.1b is the same story, which has now been worked on for half an hour by Linda, with a view to unearthing her thinking and decision-making. The bracketed comments in bold type identify the kind of thinking that underlay the actions reported. The numbers against these allow for expansion of these points in the critique beneath the narrative. The italics, interestingly, show where the original narrative was extended as a result of considering the clinical thinking that ran beneath the action and so recognizing that the full details that led up to the decisions were not included in the original narrative. It will also be noted that Linda has reshaped the written presentation in order to point up the various stages of the action and thought that she engaged in. This is indeed a matter of unpacking her implicit and tacit knowledge and thinking.

Resource 8.1b   Cancelling a patient's operation on the day of surgery (Version two)

It takes more than just knowing about the condition and being able to do the operation.

The case scenario

The context of the case
It was a Tuesday morning at 8 AM, and I arrived to review the patients on my all-day operating list. The previous Friday, I had reviewed the list, and it showed a patient with an abdominal aortic aneurysm from my vascular waiting list and two patients from the common waiting list for thyroid surgery. On the Monday, I had been working away from the Trust. Late on the previous Friday, one of the patients listed for thyroid surgery had phoned to cancel their operation because of a concurrent medical problem. In order not to miss the operating space, a patient requiring recurrent incisional hernia surgery was given the place left by the cancellation. **[1. Complex clinical problem beginning to emerge]** This new patient had been admitted to the ward on the Monday. **[2. Complex clinical problem shaping up as conflicting needs of patient, Trust, and learners]** He had been consented by the trainees ready for theatre on the Tuesday. *I recognized that overruling a decision made by learners might not be good for them, but the patient's interests had to come first. I made a mental note to talk them through this later.* **[3. Complex clinical problem is formulated as: to operate or not on the hernia patient]** *I did not make this explicit in my initial version of the narrative.*

145

I enquired why another thyroid patient had not been added, *because the type of surgery and fitness of the patient would have made for a more straightforward operation with a thyroid patient than a patient admitted with an incisional hernia. This mattered because of the length of time available on the list, the need to appraise the hernia patient of the risks, and my not having seen the hernia patient before.* I was told that this patient was next on the list. **[4a. Clinical reasoning takes account of Trust demands]** I visited the patient for the hernia repair on the ward **[4b. Clinical reasoning takes account of all that can be gained from meeting the patient]** His case notes were very thick **[4c. Clinical reasoning takes account of extent of comorbid problems]** and were being read very carefully by the consultant anaesthetist. **[4d. Clinical reasoning takes account of the concerns of other colleagues]** I observed that the patient walked with a stick **[4e. Clinical reasoning takes account of observation of patient] [5. Now the clinical solution is becoming clear – not to operate at this time – *I did not note this initially in my narrative*]**, and he told me that he was very disabled with joint problems. **[6a. Deliberation includes as a factor the priority of patient's other problems and personal story]** After a short conversation with him, it seemed to me that both he and I were less informed **[6b, c. Deliberation takes account of how the patient might be seeing his problem, and the patient's resulting needs]** than we should be about his surgical problem. This was my first knowledge of him. **[6d. Deliberation takes account of the practitioner's knowledge]** His understanding of the possible postoperative events that might complicate his recovery was very limited. **[6e. Deliberation takes account of the need to educate the patient to understand the risks and to have time to assimilate them] [7. Practical wisdom highlights the recognition of my moral responsibilities to the patient, and the need to act accordingly]**

I made the decision to postpone his case **[8a. Professional judgement]** and arranged to see him again the following Friday in my outpatient clinic **[8b. Professional judgement and agreed action plan]**. There was a feeling abroad that I was over-reacting. **[9. I now recognize overtly that there is a need to be able to explain my thinking in detail to a number of affected parties]**

Critique

Clearly, Points 1 and 2 lead up to the emergence of the complex clinical problem at Point 3. As a learner, I would expect to work on giving voice (in my head) to a more precise formulation of such problems. This problem is complex because endemic to it are competing arguments and priorities leading to different solutions.

Points 4a–e show the clinical elements considered, and the reasoning used about them. I could have said more about the logic with which I ordered these points, and as a learner would try to do so in future. Point 5 shows the clinical solution arising from these arguments. If I needed to review this solution, it would be important to be able to set out and explore the logic of my clinical reasoning.

Points 6a–e show how this clinical solution is deliberated about. They show that I recognize a number of different points of view (none of them easily prioritized), but they do not show how I go about doing this. Point 7 shows that I recognize my moral responsibilities to the patient, and respond to the patient's needs. Points 8a–b offer the professional judgement and agreed treatment plan. In Point 9, I have recognized overtly some other moral obligations that spring from this event.

A later addition

At the outpatient clinic, the patient and I had a long conversation, and I added to the information he already knew about the consequences of such surgery. He was booked for the following week, was admitted and had an uneventful operation. Postoperatively, he was cared for on the high-dependency unit. Thirty-six hours post surgery, he suffered a respiratory collapse, and a computerized tomography (CT) scan confirmed multiple pulmonary emboli. He was put on anticoagulants. Forty-eight hours later, he had a bleed into his abdominal wall, which required his emergency return to theatre and a postoperative period on the Intensive Care Unit. He subsequently made a satisfactory recovery and was discharged home. His comments about his care were that he had had a very scary time but he had felt that at all times the doctors and nurses had kept him informed and that we had had his best interests at heart. The Trust nevertheless earned a black mark for an operation cancelled on the day.

Being a surgeon daily involves far more than following protocols, doing surgery and ensuring that targets are met. In this event, I exercised a level of professional judgement which was greater than that based on a clinical decision-making strategy. Such a strategy provides a diagnosis and a plan of action to treat based on history-taking, examination and investigation. This locks the patient into a care pathway designed to result in timely and efficient treatment. This patient was inside such a process. But it was not personalized to him. It took no account of the fact that he was a high-risk patient with an uncommon and complex problem. I was perfectly capable of doing an appropriate operation, but I was not convinced it was appropriate for him.

My professional judgement resulting in my action on the day was informed by:

- my factual knowledge about the patient's condition extended by my wider exploration of it on the day (he was disabled and 'unfit' and therefore a higher risk than many – and crucially more than the thyroid case that he had replaced on the list)
- my personal knowledge of the procedural reasons why he had been added to the list at short notice and the potential mistakes that can be made through trying to 'be efficient' rather than concentrating on the specific needs of the patient
- my professional responsibility as consultant and therefore the most senior clinician managing the case, to be sure that the things that had gone on before my intervention surgically were as sound as they could be – and if they were not, to do something about it
- my previous experience in recognizing that if I felt uncomfortable about a case (even if I could not entirely explain why), I should take very careful stock of things before inflicting more injury (the operation and its subsequent consequences) on the patient
- my personal knowledge of my trainee staff, who lacked my experience and intuitive feel, who were responding to the need to fill the list, and who I felt may not have appreciated all the potential consequences of proceeding unprepared
- my ability to be able to 'break the rules' and be able to justify why
- my recognition that my responsibility was first to the patient
- my knowledge that I am morally accountable and will be held professionally answerable for the process of care of this patient
- my belief that where such a duty of care is in conflict with Trust targets, the patient's welfare must come first
- the courage to conduct myself professionally in the face of pressures to conform.

Note
This scenario brings together details of a story that first appeared in part in de Cossart and Fish (2005, pp. 171–3) and in part in Fish and Coles (2005, pp. 86–8).

This resource, then, offers both one way of learning to pinpoint the professional judgements made in a case and to explore them, and also two ways of annotating the case to include these new insights. The following resource offers a very different way of identifying the points at which personal professional judgement has been exercised.

RESOURCE 8.2: CLARIFYING THE PLACE OF PERSONAL PROFESSIONAL JUDGEMENT

Resource 8.2 table offers a generalized list of the five main processes that the doctor engages in throughout the Clinical Thinking Pathway, and upon which he/she brings to bear his or her personal professional judgements.

We can see from Resource 8.2 that the first two columns identify the processes of the Clinical Thinking Pathway, and the third indicates the detailed thinking associated with them. The final column shows how the doctor may use personal professional judgement to weigh up, prioritize or discard elements of the evidence available, as not significant in coming to a final decision.

This resource can be used to reinforce understanding about what is involved in personal professional judgement, and its major significance in getting the treatment right for the patient. But it can also be used to help a learner map a particular case using this format.

RESOURCE 8.3: EXPLORING THE QUALITY OF BOTH FORMS OF JUDGEMENT

By contrast, Resource 8.3 provides learners with a means of recognizing the quality of both forms of their judgements. Here, every column offers an important commentary on the judgement and what has led up to it. Again, this can only be used in relation to a given case, and the best evidence of progress will, of course, come from a pattern across cases (taking account of complexity of case and level and stage of career).

In this resource, the first column shows that a hasty or unquestioned, habitual judgement will place the doctor in a discrete category of 'unsatisfactory' (which must be retrieved before real development can occur). All other judgements that have been arrived at through some intelligent and conscious thinking offer promise of progress on a developmental continuum that rises from self-interested decisions to wise judgements. Wise judgement is clearly the aim, but even the most senior doctors may begin the process of formulating a judgement by starting with self-interest, which they then override for reasons we shall see below.

The second column offers in more detail the motivations that lie behind these judgements. It shows that the unsatisfactory judgement is made when the doctor is not motivated to weigh up the complexity of choices available, but merely 'goes through the motions' of being a doctor. The developing doctor, on the other hand, is seen moving through a continuum from concern only for their own self-interest, to a real understanding of what is involved in putting the patient first. That is, the doctor moves from concern only with self and the impression made by good performance; through a stage where it begins to be clearer what is involved in putting patient first, while still clinging conservatively to the preservation of self-esteem; and finally reaches an understanding that genuinely valuing the patient involves transcending all concern for self (see Chapter 9 for more detail on this).

Resource 8.2 Clarifying the personal professional judgements made during the Clinical Thinking Pathway

Processes	Overall activity	Detail	Personal professional judgements to be made
Process 1 Formulate the case	• Collect the evidence	• Observe patient • Converse and establish rapport with patient • Take patient's history • Listen to patient narrative, focusing on key issues • Examine patient • Appropriately investigate patient • Communicate with other relevant people	• The validity and reliability of information provided by others at all points • When sufficient information has been collected • Relevance of own values and humanity as they relate to the case
Process 2 Work over the evidence within the clinical reasoning section	• Identify the salient factors in Process 1 • Distil the meaning of the clinical evidence	Identify and draw on: • the salient factors in the case • all relevant propositional knowledge • research findings where relevant • experiential knowledge • contextual information about the patient and their inter-dependents • familiarity with the Trust as an organization and its requirements and resources	• What are the salient factors? • The quality of interpretations being offered by others • Relevance of information provided • Risks and benefits of different choices • How widely should patterns be sought? • Differentiating between opinions and knowledge

Process 3 Receive/review clinical solution(s)	• Come to a clinical decision/conclusion/reconsider it	• Identify main problem • Determine a working hypothesis • Make a working diagnosis • Make a plan for care • Defend decision	• Recognizing the solution as generally the right thing to do • Critiquing that decision in terms of appropriateness for patient
Process 4 Engage in the deliberative part of the pathway	• List the key issues and pressures on the decision about what is right for the patient	Consider issues related to: • patient and supporters • patient's moral and ethical needs • all that I as doctor bring • what the Trust requires • what my profession, and society require • what the law requires • the demands of the unexpected additional issue(s)	• Prioritizing the list • Choosing between competing demands • Allowing for the ambiguities of the particular case • Listening to own intuitions • Discounting own interests
Process 5 Come to a professional judgement about wise action	• Design a treatment plan in the light of the clinical decision	• Re-assess treatment criteria • Choose between alternative treatments • Provide relief or deal with cause • Consider short- and long-term management.	• Critiquing the decision • Recognizing the need for periodic reconsideration of treatment plan

Resource 8.3 Process and product professional judgements differentiated (to be used in respect of individual cases – remembering that all cases are context-specific)

Kind of professional judgement (leading to:)	Response to patient case	Motivation (where the doctor places self in relation to managing the patient)	Questions learner asked themselves	Questions/instructions from teacher to learner	New agenda for learner
Wise judgement (enlightenment growing)	• Sees each case as needing to be enquired into beyond the obvious, defines what is needed for the best for the patient, can do/obtain what is needed (checks with senior as appropriate), then does it. Can make rational sense out of intuitive judgement and use pathway both ways up • Treats all judgements as potentially provisional and requiring revisiting	• Willing and able to put patient's interests first at all times in decision-making, even if this risks own interests and position in some way	• How can I achieve what is best for the patient? • What else should be deliberated upon? • Who else should I talk to beyond the obvious team?	• Think about the range of people to unpack your thinking with. What have you learnt about yourself and how might you develop further?	• Use the clinical thinking pathway for increasingly complex cases

Maturing judgement (developing insight)	• Open-minded to the complexity of each case; builds on experience. Has a proper respect for conservative management, but beginning to balance safety of patient with carefully judged risks	• Beginning to put patient first in decision-making, but still lacks experience to step outside own needs in favour of patient's interests. Beginning to see that one can play it too safe	• What should I take into account here? • Should I discuss this with my senior?	• Could you try some clinical reflective writing on specific cases, aimed at exploring your professional judgements?	• Refine your clinical thinking by presenting cases starting with the professional judgements you have made
Self-interested judgement (need for considerable developmental work)	• Selects tactics known to please; closed minded about choices. Chooses what fits limited experience rather than seeing the wider context	• Choice of decisions and resultant behaviour designed to enhance own performance and achievements in eyes of consultant	• What would my seniors do and how can I please them? • What am I personally able do in this case, and how will I do that?	• How can I help you better to explore and use the Clinical Thinking Pathway – perhaps we need more discussion together?	• Need to use Clinical Thinking Pathway in a number of cases under close supervision
Hasty/habitual judgement (recognition that this is unsatisfactory)	• Knee-jerk reaction/going through the motions unthinkingly	• Has not even considered that choices are available	• None • I've seen this before, haven't I? Why shouldn't I do the same again?	• Please think about why you made that decision and explore and explain the logic behind it	• Can retrieve this by beginning to explore the Clinical Thinking Pathway and using it appropriately

Developing the Wise Doctor

Wise judgement, then, which is something to aspire to, involves balancing reason and emotion in sensing what is best for the patient, gaining a disinterested (detached) interest in the patient, standing up for whatever is best for the patient, and taking a temperate course that is aimed first and foremost at the conquest of the patient's suffering. There is no room here for the arrogant voices of self-preservation, self-concern, self-interest: only for genuine humility, which, as TS Eliot points out, 'is endless', and which should not be confused with unctuous claims to being 'humble'. (We shall explore this in more detail in the following chapter.)

Column three then characterizes the response to the patient that springs from these motivations, and column four offers the doctor examples of the kinds of questions they might ask themselves at points along this continuum. Column five indicates the kind of things that teachers might say to the learning doctor at various points, and column six indicates some ways forward. This final column provides some possibilities for an agenda that would be best set by the *learner*, rather than the teacher.

Readers are invited to use this resource to explore and discuss the quality of their judgements and, for the sake of patients, to raise their aspirations in respect of them, even if the ultimate attainment of wise judgements seems a long way off!

END-NOTES

We leave readers with two final subsections. Firstly, we offer a caveat that applies to both this chapter and the previous one. Secondly, we offer a closing scenario and commentary.

In attempting to make very clear both the elements of clinical thinking and how to explore professional judgement, we have inevitably simplified a number of things. Of these, we have already warned of the dangers of the reductionism that models bring. We now issue a warning about the need to use these processes in more complex ways. The helicoid is a reminder that thinking may need to spiral up and down the elements presented in linear form. The following is a reminder of the need to consider all thinking and judgements as eternally provisional.

Caveat: The importance of revisiting decisions and thinking at all stages

We have presented the pathways as leading doctors directly to clear judgements, but would strongly emphasize the fact that in real practice, clinicians will always go back over the pathway and revisit the decisions and the thinking that led to them. This is particularly so when elements that do not fit emerge and are faced squarely. Indeed, as a general rule, we would say: where at any stage uncertainty remains about the accuracy of diagnosis, recycling through the pathway must always be carried out.

Demonstrating the quality of the doctor's professional judgements

The following example illustrates this.

Scenario

A 28-year-old male presents to the acute hospital A & E department on Christmas Day. His symptoms are of acute pain in both calves, he is unable to walk and feels extremely unwell. Clinical examination reveals hypotension, thin thready pulses, upper-limb peripheral cyanosis, tense calves, impalpable pulses in the feet but with capilliary return in the toes. On receiving the blood results, which demonstrate acidosis and renal failure, and urine demonstrating rhabdomyosis, a diagnosis of acute renal failure and bilateral calf compression syndrome is made. The precise initiating cause of this at this point is unclear. Steps are put in place to begin treatment of the renal failure, initiating renal dialysis, and arrangements are made to decompress the muscle compartments in both calves.

Twelve hours later, his condition has deteriorated further, and further clinical reasoning takes place to reframe the problem and to continue to find an initial cause. There is developing a strong intuitive sense (based on experience) that his heart may be the primary dysfunctional organ. There is a strong need for the clinicians to hold open the final framing of the clinical problem, and to continue to revise their clinical reasoning, alongside further investigations. These include, in addition to blood tests and clinical monitoring, ultrasound imaging of the heart and peripheral vessels.

Here, then is an example of the kinds of 'shifting sands' in the development of a patient's problems and needs. These require willingness to rethink the decisions, and result in many revisits to the pathway and various readjustments to the decisions made.

Finally, we offer the following closing scenario as a further example of how learners and teachers might use these resources. As you read this, you are invited to pinpoint the teaching strategies used here.

Final scenario: the educational meeting the morning after

Cons: Right ... Well done all of you, for getting here and for having a go at the task. We'll take long enough to explore properly what you have come up with. This is an entirely private meeting, so feel free to say what you like. I think it's going to be interesting ... We're all here to learn. ... So ... OK Michael, why don't you kick off for us.

Michael: Yes ... well, thank you ... I used the table (Exploring the Quality of my judgements) to make my own version. Here is a copy ... I've tried to set down my involvement and the kinds of decisions that I made. [*Offers table below. Consultant says 'Ah, good'. Michael talks table through*]

What I did	The kinds of professional judgement I used
In ward saw patient, and having reviewed the results made a judgement that he needed an operation	Wise judgement
Talked to patient about what we would do. Discussed possibility of colostomy but said it would depend on what we found. Checked it out with Mrs C. She agreed	Provisional judgement (wise judgement) or perhaps maturing judgement
Performed the operation in standard fashion. Found that resection was possible but also thought anastomosis was feasible. Discussed with anaesthetist because patient was pretty sick. We agreed that short procedure was the most appropriate	Maturing, to wise judgement. Made a decision, reviewed it and discussed with other relevant colleagues
Allowed SpR1 to close the wound whilst I organized bed in HDU	Wise judgement based on my personal experience of working with SpR1

[*Michael finishes talking the table through, and there is silence . He then continues as follows.*]

... Actually, I was challenged by the SpR on the other colorectal unit, who seemed to think that I should have done an anastomosis ... But I think he might have been demonstrating self-interested judgement. I would want to argue that I showed wise professional judgement in this case, but I don't know what the rest of you think.

[*The consultant allows silence and space for the other two doctors (John and Jane) to comment and ask questions ... Only when they have finished does she continue:*]

Cons: Thank you very much, Michael. I must say I believe you put the patient at the heart of this case and did override what might have been a 'peer challenge' to do an anastomosis. Well done. You revisited your decision and used others to add further to what was your final definitive judgement to do a colostomy. I agree with your self-assessment here. Now: what did you learn from doing this exercise?

Michael: Well, a surprising amount. At first I thought it was a strange exercise ... but I had a go ... And then I began to realize just how many more resources I'd tapped into in getting to the final professional judgement. So ... yes, it's quite interesting. I shall use it again.

Cons: OK. Now come on John, you go next. I particularly asked you to think about what judgements you made when you were examining Mr Murray in front of me.

John: Well, I'm afraid that though I've got my own notes, I haven't made any for any of you.

Cons: No problem ... just go ahead and talk us through.

John: Well, I was conscious that you were watching and so I tried to do the examination by the book.

Cons: Yes and you did do the examination well. But ... Would anyone else like to offer a comment?

Michael: I'd ask: what sort of judgement you think that was? [*Cons nods*]

John: Well I guess I was in self-interested judgement mode. I was keen to get it right for me – that's not to say I did not have the patient's best interests at heart, but I did want to be seen to do well.

Jane: Well, I thought that was what a consultant was looking for when we are asked to examine a patient.

Cons: Well, ... so what are you *now* thinking, about that?

Jane: Um ... I think that the more inexperienced you are the more your mind is on getting the examination right and to impress. ... But ... well ... I'd never thought before that that might be in conflict with the patient's best interests. ...

John: Yes ... It's such an easy phrase, isn't it 'putting the patient first'? ... I suppose we all just assume that we automatically do that by just being there, but perhaps there is more to it than that.

Michael: I think I've learnt that I need to be more careful about how I judge Foundation doctors when they examine in front of me. ...

Brief commentary

The opening words here set a private and therefore safe environment in which learners can explore frankly the results of their work. The choice of doctor to begin this exploration is interesting. Jane is the only woman of the three learners, but the teacher picks the two men, choosing the senior first, and then the most junior. Perhaps she knows that Jane, though the middle-level doctor, is the weakest at self-critique.

The teacher also sustains this encouraging environment, by not chiding John for bringing no paperwork. But this does not lower the standard she expects, because she has already praised Michael for his table.

The strategies used to draw the learners to think deeply about their practice and to share this thinking aloud are *silence* and *space*! In not coming in first with an evaluative comment, but holding back and waiting to see what sense the others have made of this, the teacher learns more about what the learners need from her. Indeed, she speaks the least of all, and because she stands back, gradually the learners begin to say, and to think, more. They even challenge their own previous thoughts and assumptions. But, when she does speak, she uses her time profitably in appreciating what they have achieved, and not labouring what they have already grasped.

In all this, she offers a good model.

FURTHER READING

de Cossart L, Fish D (2005) *Cultivating a Thinking Surgeon: New Perspectives on Clinical Teaching, Learning and Assessment*. Shrewsbury: tfm Publications: Chapter 8. [This chapter offers illustrations of how professional judgement can be explored, though it provides a less refined version of Resource 8.2 above.]

Montgomery K (2006) *How Doctors Think: Clinical Judgement and the Practice of Medicine*. Oxford: Oxford University Press: Chapter 3. [This important chapter explores the humanistic qualities of professional judgement.]

9

The therapeutic relationship of wise doctor and valued patient: Bringing the core together

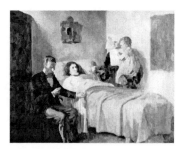

The following is slightly adapted from a handwritten letter actually received by a consultant from a patient, following a consultation. The consultant filed it as a resource for teaching. You are invited to read this chapter with this letter in mind.

Dear Dr Morgan,

I wanted to write to say thank you for putting my mind at rest yesterday. I know that I must have taken up a lot of your time but I feel much better today and I am going to see my own doctor tomorrow.

Ever since my cancer surgery I have been given the best of care but I did not seem to be able to get an answer to my question about why I was still feeling so weak and tired. It is three months now since the operation and I still cannot go to the supermarket. I am not sleeping properly and my own doctor had suggested some sleeping tablets but I am not a tablet taker and do not want to start now. Everyone has been very kind.

I have been quite sure that there was something that was being hidden from me and that I was really not going to get better. My friend's husband, who had a similar operation just before me, is back to normal. In fact they have just been on a round the world trip. Living alone is hard and since my husband died I have not been right. I feel so awful at not being able to cope.

I think you are right, the results of all the tests are fine. I need to accept some help at home and get my life into routine again. I will see you in six months at my next routine visit.

Please give the nurses in the clinic and the rest of your team my thanks.

Yours sincerely,

Mary Thomas

Questions to ask yourself whilst reading this chapter
1. What does a patient want from a doctor?
2. What makes for a good relationship with a patient?
3. What is my role in relation to each patient?
4. How do the invisibles affect such a relationship?
5. How do I decide what is best for the patient?
6. What motivates me in making a relationship with a patient?

INTRODUCTION

In the last five chapters, we have explored the elements we believe to be at the core of medicine. These are what we have called 'the invisibles' because they are either implicit or tacit aspects of the doctor's practice. The invisibles are: the significance of the context of the patient case; the professionalism of the doctor; the forms of knowledge the doctor uses; the clinical thinking the doctor engages in; and the professional judgements the doctor makes. Each needs careful consideration by the learning doctor, and will repay individual exploration, as we have seen. But none of these elements of practice is intended, ultimately, to be treated separately. They need to come together in a wise doctor who can harness consideration of them all in providing for the best interests of the patient. In this chapter, we argue that what determines the quality of patient care is *how* and *why* these invisibles (both separately and as a whole) are drawn on by the doctor.

This involves both reminding teachers about – and also making explicit for learners' consideration – the arguments for a way of practising medicine that we fear is becoming all but lost in the current demands of the Western world. It is a way of practising that, though still subscribed to privately by doctors, seems to have been officially ditched in the present restrictive climate, with its materialistic, rule-bound, contract-governed, distrust-focused approach to 'managing' patients.

The practice of medicine that we are commending here is about a less calculating and more humanistic approach to patient care. But it is not 'soft'. Indeed, it is highly demanding and can only be achieved at a real cost to the doctor. We characterize it as 'a therapeutic relationship' between doctor and patient. By 'the therapeutic relationship' we mean something special about the way the doctor meets the patient. The term makes a statement about the quality of time spent with the patient (as opposed to the length) because the patient has had what he/she needs and has been met by the doctor more than halfway. This is partly about the patient feeling nurtured irrespective of whether they can be cured, irrespective of the doctor's technical skills, and *even* irrespective of the doctor's apparently brusque surface manner, provided that beneath that surface the doctor has 'a heart of gold'.

Doctors need to come to an informed view about what kind of relationship with patients they should strive for. Their ability to create nurturing relationships (or not) with their patients will shape their whole professional life, making it meaningful or leaving it devoid of something inexpressible yet significant. Further, whether or not doctors are consciously aware of it, their work daily expresses how they see patients in relation to themselves, and patients in turn are highly skilled at recognizing this.

The content of this chapter will be challenging, even uncomfortable, for some readers, but we do not apologize for this. The cutting edge of education is not designed for comfort but for disturbing our ideas, raising awkward questions, and thinking daring thoughts. Doctors, who as practitioners daily engage in hard tasks, and meet difficult decisions and life in the raw, inevitably, as professionals, also face periodic challenges to their most cherished ideas and ideals. They need to be equipped to discuss, reconsider and, where appropriate, defend them.

We offer this chapter, then, in the spirit of confronting learning doctors with some demanding ideas to consider, and some language that will help them to respond to these. For us, the wise doctor is one who will have penetrated the surface of the invisibles, and will have recognized and learnt to live with the ambiguities and complexities as well as the incompleteness and unpredictability of medicine. But we would also want such a doctor to be able to establish a restorative and caring relationship with patients. This is a relationship that, while it may not be able to cure, can heal, and that invites the needy patient into a relationship that enriches both carer and cared for alike (Campbell, 1984, p. 107).

This chapter is divided into five parts. The first section offers and explores the heuristic, which is designed to prompt readers to think about the doctor/patient relationship, and highlights some key issues for consideration. Secondly, the invisibles we have already explored are reconsidered in the light of how they might influence the doctor/patient relationship. The third section explores a more holistic approach to the relationship, in which the invisible elements so far considered are brought together for the sake of the patient. This alerts us to some new invisibles – the moral and ethical conflicts and ambiguities that bubble beneath the surface of medical practice in respect of how doctors relate to patients. The fourth section offers some learning resources designed to help readers discuss the practical implications of the chapter. The final section of this chapter will then consider briefly how similar to the 'therapeutic relationship' of the wise doctor and valued patient is the 'pedagogic relationship' of wise teacher and valued learner.

Note

It should be noted that when we searched the literature, seeking help in making explicit the complexities of what we were already thinking of as the therapeutic relationship (looking, for example, at the writings of Berger, Heath and Balint, who interestingly are all GPs), the text that most helped us was Campbell's *Moderated Love: A Theology of Professional Care*. We therefore acknowledge with gratitude that our expression of much of the following content is heavily influenced by Campbell's language. Because his ideas struck such a chord with us, we have subjected them to careful critical scrutiny, and have somewhat reluctantly eschewed the very specifically Christian language Campbell uses, because by no means every reader will share this. We do believe, however, that the more generally spiritual ideas captured by Cambell's phrase 'the secular sacrament of medical care' are vital in medicine and are far more ubiquitous than is realized. These we use without apology. It follows that any errors of logic and exposition in the following are ours and not Campbell's.

THE DOCTOR/PATIENT RELATIONSHIP

We offer the painting shown in Figure 9.1 as a prompt to enable doctors to begin to think more deeply about the doctor/patient relationship. We offer the picture before the commentary on it, so that readers can form their own impression of it

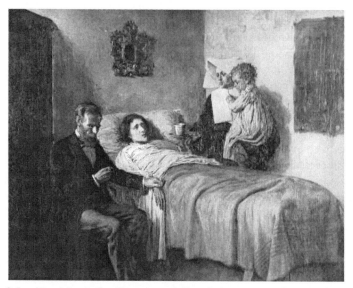

Figure 9.1   Heuristic 6: the Picasso painting *Science and Charity* (Barcelona, early 1897. Oil on canvas, 197 cm × 249.5 cm. Barcelona, Museu Picasso).

first. The commentary that follows is offered by Linda de Cossart. We then use this to open up some key issues that the rest of the chapter will explore.

A personal commentary

A print of this painting, *Science and Charity*, by Pablo Picasso has hung on my office wall for many years. I was most struck by it on a visit to the Picasso museum in Barcelona – firstly, because it was so unlike any other painting by Picasso that I had seen, and, secondly, because it spoke out to me (and still does) about the subtleties of our relationship with patients and their loved ones and how this relationship is an abiding link through generations of members of the profession of medicine.

Picasso puts the patient at the centre of the picture. The tragic expression on the woman's face suggests to me that she is going to die. The doctor portrays a serious expression, as he sits thoughtfully taking her pulse. I see this as the outward appearance of an experienced and sensitive practitioner who is preparing himself in his mind to share with the family the hopelessness of the case. His act of touching the patient conveys the importance of physical contact with a patient – in this case by a very common clinical assessment, recording the pulse. This act, I believe, allows him both to confirm his clinical impression, to ensure the patient knows he is there, and to indicate to those around him his concern for the patient. I also see in this act his making time for himself, to be sure his assessment is right and creating a few moments in which to gather together his thoughts. He is in no hurry. He is, after all, seated. In this seated position, he is at the same level as the patient, leaving the others to look down on them. He is not the dominant figure in this scene. That is left to the patient.

But there is an element in the painting that is inconsistent with the idea that the woman is dying. The nun is holding out to her a cup. The reader is left to assume what is in it. The gesture is that of 'offering a cup of water', but equally it could be warm milk (it is probably not tea, as the décor indicates a Spanish style of furniture as well as the habit of the nun being more likely to belong to a Southern European order). But if the woman is dying, this seems inappropriate. Surely, as an experienced nun, this lady knows the score, knows it is too late.

It is interesting to note that this reaching out is the only movement in an otherwise totally static picture. One is left wondering about its significance, whether it is merely a compositional device to prevent a totally static picture, or whether there was some other motivation to include it.

I have delved deeper into the mind of the painter while writing this, in order to offer another possible explanation. Picasso was 16 when he painted this prize-winning picture. It is perhaps not what one might expect from such a young man. But three years before he had watched his eight-year-old sister die. It is reported that sitting at the end of her bed, he prayed to God to let her live, promising to give up painting if this would happen. But she died. Perhaps, then, including the cup indicates the frailty of the painter (who is also, in a sense, standing near the bedside) and who is seeking comfort and hope even in the face of death by including it in the painting.

In this painting, Picasso has demonstrated superb talent and used it to emphasize the role of the doctor and the reliance of others on him. The doctor is gently taking in the context and examining the patient. We can only imagine the rest. The inclusion of a child at the bedside of the dying woman is rather modern by the standards of the day. Again, I believe that perhaps this is Picasso indicating to us the importance of not excluding important members of the family.

Clearly, I have brought to this commentary my values and ideas about medical practice, and they have shaped how I see the doctor and the whole scene. I have offered an interpretation (in respect of what is in the painting and what it might all mean) and defended that interpretation by reference to both what is in the painting and some facts about Picasso, which I gained through researching the painting. I have added my own insights into why he might have painted the nurse offering the cup of milk or water.

Some key issues for consideration

Patients are vulnerable. No matter how much they know about themselves, their symptoms and sometimes their diagnosis, they have to have doctors to confirm their disease, to offer them treatment and to provide 'more than a presence but skill, and not just personal concern but highly disciplined services targeted on specific needs' (William F May, quoted in Campbell, 1984, p. 92).

However strong patients are in their suffering, it usually reduces their stamina and weakens their belief in themselves. By contrast, doctors are powerful in, and as result of, their skills and knowledge; they have the physical strength and staying power of the fit; and they are highly motivated to cure, improve or, at minimum, palliate, the sick. But their sense that they can almost always improve the lot of the patient can seduce doctors into enjoying the exercise of their power.

There is, as Campbell so wisely pointed out, an odd juxtaposition between 'service and personal advantage'. Can the doctor claim both at the same time? Or is there a slight but significant balance to be kept between caring as a selfless service to others (insofar as we humanly can) and caring for the sick as a means of being – or of demonstrating that one is – virtuous. (And is one being 'virtuous' for the sake of the patient or for the privilege and power that virtue brings?) This is a version of the point TS Eliot makes in *Murder in the Cathedral* (near the end of Part One), when he labels 'the right deed for the wrong reason' as the 'greatest form of treason'.

What this reveals is that the *motivation* beneath action (the invisible reasons why doctors behave as they do, which are driven by values or ethical principles) is what determines the wise doctor and shapes the quality of the relationship with the patient. As Johnson (1990, pp.154–5) points out, 'motivation does matter enormously ...' but 'motives alone are not enough'. Motives and ethical principles must go together in the same way that its engine powers a car along a certain road. And, as we shall see, in the end there can be no fudging the choices.

Diverging paths do not permit compromise, *syncretism* (the policy of holding on to two different views rather than make a decision between them) is flawed (Johnson, 1990, pp. 85–6).

How then, does all this relate to the invisibles we have explored so far?

THE INVISIBLES AND THE DOCTOR/PATIENT RELATIONSHIP

The invisibles that we have explored so far as important elements of medical practice now need to be explored individually in terms of the motivation behind using them on behalf of the patient and the purpose behind bringing them together for the care of the patient.

Having encouraged learning doctors to be more alert to the invisibles, we must now lead them to ask: For what purpose am I to consider them? What is their ultimate individual significance in relation to the care of the patient? This will then provide the basis for exploring the attitude with which the invisibles will be drawn upon holistically in the service of the patient.

The invisibles examined individually for motivation

The following brief re-examination of the invisibles involves raising questions about the doctor's attitudes and motivations in respect of them. This is designed to reveal the complexity and ambiguity of what drives the doctor, and will ultimately lead us to consider these same motivations at the heart of the relationships that the doctor makes with the patient and that the teacher makes with the learner.

Context

We argued earlier that careful attention to and interpretation of the context in which the patient presents is a vital aspect of getting patient care 'right'. But we now ask whether in attending to the context, the doctor shows an attitude of 'hubris' (overconfidence or arrogance – which the Greeks saw as inviting disaster or ruin); of humility (a kind of personal, unpretentious modesty, which puts others first but should not be confused with abasing oneself); or some odd and illogical mixture of the two. And beneath the prevailing attitude here will be the prevailing motivation(s) and ethical principles. Does the doctor attend to the context for his/her own glory and self-importance, for the sake of the patient, or for mixed motives – in which case, how are these balanced? And what view of this balance does the doctor have (for example, that it is inevitable, regrettable or of no account)?

Professionalism

Similarly, in refining ideas about, and seeking to extend, their professionalism, will doctors be grounding their personal development in the ideal of gaining position and privilege, in the ideal of striving to serve the patient and offer them unconditional regard as having unique human value, or in an ambiguous mixture of these (and in what proportions)? And how far does this matter to the doctor?

Knowledge

In considering the range of forms of knowledge the doctor brings to the patient's case, is that knowledge seen by the doctor as bolstering his/her credibility and personal power or as a means to come to know the patient in order to come to know that which is even more important – what is best for the patient? Or, again, might there be a mixture of these? How are these kinds of knowledge balanced by the doctor, and what does this say finally about his/her values in relating to the patient?

Clinical thinking

If we are right that the quality of the doctor's clinical thinking is in the rigour with which he/she exercises the elements of the pathway we have described, then for whose sake is the doctor being rigorous: for his/her own sake, for the patient's, or for a mixture? And, again, how is the mixture balanced?

Professional judgements

Does the quality of the professional judgements reached deserve the accolade 'wise' only when the doctor has transcended self-interest? Or can this never happen? Is it an unattainable ideal?

We offer a summary of these ideas in Figure 9.2.

The invisibles brought together: for what purpose?

All this, of course, raises questions about the attitude with which this core of medicine (the invisibles), is drawn upon as a whole in the care of the patient. It also raises wider issues: for example, about whether altruistic motivation is ever possible; whether self-importance is inevitably the unquenchable victor over true virtue; whether self-advancement will always outweigh 'disinterested' care, which is 'the impossible ideal' that recognizes full value in every individual, however damaged, however oppressed, however bereft of hope (Campbell, 1984, p. 85).

Campbell persuasively argues that altruism, for all its complexity, is entirely appropriate to, and necessary for, 'professional helping'. He concedes that it is elusive and perhaps possible only as an ideal commitment, which is 'frequently not honoured'. He says: '... We must recognize that its requirements are more than can be reasonably expected' (Campbell, 1984, p. 83). But, we would argue, they are a light in the dark world of dumbed-down expectations and deliberately lowered 'standards', which emanate from the confusion of equality with equity.

It should be noted that in what follows we are not seeking the one definitive

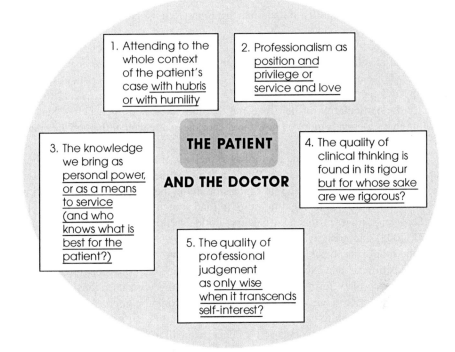

Figure 9.2 The key elements at the core of medicine and their significance.

answer or solution to the issues raised. Rather, we are providing fuel to enable doctors to confront and challenge or refine their own vision of the doctor/patient relationship, in the belief that a wise doctor attains and then retains his/her wisdom *only* for so long as he/she recognizes the ambiguities at the heart of medical practice. This is because, of course (as Campbell helpfully points out), 'no human acts are wholly disinterested', but there is a difference between activities that are *only* self-seeking, and those where a claim can be made to concern for others (Campbell, 1984, pp. 6–7).

WHAT IS INVOLVED IN THE THERAPEUTIC RELATIONSHIP?

Doctors are familiar with the patient's utterance: 'there is no more they can do for me … I've been discharged'. When this happens, the relationship has foundered and healthcare has failed. By contrast, Montgomery (2006, p. 162) says that when the doctor/patient relationship goes well it is *'one of the triumphs of human society'*. But it is a triumph only when the relationship has at its heart the plight of the sick patient, not just the cure of the disease. Cure of the disease is of course an essential element of the doctor's role, but, as is so often the case, cure is not always possible. Cure might be described as the bonus in the relationship and to be handled with humility rather than triumph. If it is possible, it makes the doctor's job so much easier.

We reserve the term 'therapeutic' (which is not one that Campbell uses) for the very special relationship that indicates the mutual *working together* of a wise doctor who brings a range of qualities (as examined below) and a patient who is willing not merely to meet the doctor, but where appropriate to reveal to the doctor the particularity of their case and the individuality of their being. Such a 'willingness' depends more on how the doctor meets the patient than on the character of the patient.

In order to achieve this, the doctor has to pick his or her way through a number of complexities and ambiguities. Wisdom is not gained overnight. Neither is it without cost. But, wisdom and its expression in the therapeutic relationship with a patient does provide an ideal to aspire to (and sometimes to reach). And that is perhaps, important, in this 21st century world of 'liquid modernity' (Bauman, 2000, 2005) and 'risk aversion' (Neuberger, 2005). As Fish and Higgs (2007) say, the role of responsible members of a profession, 'is precisely to argue their moral position, ... and exercise their clinical thinking and professional judgement in the service of differing individuals, while making wise decisions about the relationship between individuals' privacy and the common good'.

Such an approach to care involves a commitment to each patient that (though not limitless) certainly involves active concern, a will to work with rather than on the ill person, and a kind of open-ended helpfulness (Campbell, 1984, p.104). This, we believe, requires balancing commitment to the patient, to all other patients and to a duty to self. In addition to the knowledge and skill doctors have, they must 'profess' the following: service to mankind; disinterested love (a valuing of the other that takes full interest in them, without personal gain of any kind – including seeking a reputation for wisdom); and respect for every person's dignity and rights. They must also promise consistency of care, which means *both* continuity of care *and* a high standard of care.

This personal commitment cannot be captured solely in the current language of the 'contract'. It is a relationship that goes beyond 'codes of conduct' or guarantees of trustworthiness as safeguarded by professional codes of ethics and the disciplining of those whose conduct lies outside the acceptable. Campbell (1984, p. 104) offers instead the term 'covenant', which avoids calculation and which promises active concern and involves altruistic motivation and the earning of trust. But none of this is straightforward. O'Neill (2002, p. 69) has pointed out that, ironically, 'Our clearest images of trust do not link it to openness and transparency at all ... Mutual respect *precludes* rather than *requires* across-the-board openness between doctor and patient ...'

This warns us, then, that at the heart of being a wise doctor is a judicious balancing of the following: the demands made on him or her; the motivations and ethical principles that a doctor brings to his/her practice; and the doctor's ability to recognize, navigate through and resolve (temporarily) the ambiguities inherent in serving another. The rest of this section looks in more detail at these.

The relationship of the carer and cared for

Campbell (1984, p. 15) suggests that 'professional care is one possible response to the fragmentation of our world, which expresses itself in illness and many other forms of social distress'. He argues that 'the person who offers professional care seeks (perhaps unknowingly) to restore that lost unity, yet also inevitably shares in the fragmentation'. But he also points out that there are anomalies and ambiguities even in attempts to 'do good'. He lists as appropriate and necessary attitudes for those who aspire to care: 'penitence, hope, realism and a search for lost harmony'.

Campbell (1984, p. 16) quotes Ruth Wilkes on 'the basic orientation required by those who make it their occupation to help others'. She writes (Wilkes, 1981, p. 62):

> 'It is an approach that calls for humility, patience, an attitude of respect towards the world, and an awareness of its infinite mystery and complexity. This way of helping is difficult because it requires a detachment that does not come naturally. The inclination in any relationship is always to meddle ... If, however, we can detach ourselves from other people in an attitude of non-possessive concern, we leave them free to change in their own way ...'

There is need for rationality and detachment in professional work, which is caught in the term 'disinterested concern' (interest in the other without seeking gain). But there is a danger even here. The *seeming* altruism of patronizing professionals 'is a luxury they can afford, when there is no real challenge to their status, professional privilege and material security in acting in this manner'. By contrast, genuinely disinterested concern is manifest only when there is real cost to the self in expressing it (Campbell, 1984, pp. 11–12). This is a reaching out to each patient (however difficult) in the desire to enhance that other person's value by providing attentive care, in a non-judgemental way that increases the other's self-esteem, and which ironically also can reduce anxious demand. This involves doctors 'spending themselves'.

Such a reaching out requires the non-rational connection that feeling alone can create. But the doctor cannot abandon his knowledge and skill. Thus, we employ the professional helper to maintain this balance of reason and emotion (Campbell, 1984, p. 88). In this context, the title of the Picasso painting (*Science and Charity*) is perhaps germane. Medicine contains both, using the original meaning of charity as 'disinterested love'.

What, then, is the texture of this relationship really like? It is far from the 'weeping with one's patient' advocated by some in earlier days. It is more complex than the empathy and compassion that are so often used to wrap up and commend a whole bundle of attitudes. There should be hard-headedness and consistency in the care offered, unlike the more erratic and turbulent attempts to help that emanate from family and friends. In the ideal, at least, the climate of professional help is always a moderate one, temperate and without extremes and sudden changes. To some extent, the term 'closeness' to the patient is useful. But what does this mean?

Developing the Wise Doctor

Closeness to the patient

The phrase 'therapeutic relationship' suggests a closeness to the patient. But we do not believe that it is well summed up in the popular terms 'empathy' and 'compassion'. Rather, we see it as involving mutuality, identification, intimacy and discipline. As we shall see, these are tightly interrelated concepts.

We accept both that the professional who cannot participate in the other's feeling (empathy) is too distant to help, and also that where loss of self occurs as a result of identification with the patient, there is too much closeness for professional help. With Campbell (1984, p. 82), we see that 'it is in the control of sympathy that the importance of the professional ethos may again be seen' (as, for example, in not voicing natural reactions to squalor, degradation, mutilation). And we recognize that 'empathy' is not what it is about because it is possible to go through the motions of empathy.

Paraphrasing Pellegrino and Thomasma, who are quoted by Campbell, we would argue that a therapeutic relationship is one of mutual consent, which achieves the well-being of the patient (and therefore the doctor) 'by working in, with and through the body'. As Campbell points out, the reference here to the bodies of both the doctor and patient identifies the unique feature of medical acts as bodily relationships (Campbell, 1984, p. 28). He dismisses the 'sentimental existentialist' idea that it is enough to "be present" to one another, because in a crisis, the ill person needs "not simply presence" but skill, not just personal concern but highly disciplined services targeted on specific needs' (Campbell, 1984, p. 92)

The success of the therapeutic relationship probably relies on the patient's revelation of an inner world of experience, to which there is no access from outside, except so far as the other person chooses to grant it, and which achieves an echoing response in the doctor. We would go beyond Campbell here and suggest that this 'revelation' by the patient, which is met halfway by the doctor, allows the pair to make meaning (sense) of the patient's needs as it were 'in the air between them' (which means that neither one has the 'key' to those needs, but that they must collaborate orally together in order to reach an understanding).

Thus, while avoiding being patronizing, the doctor must get close to the individuality of the patient through an awareness of common humanity and of mutual dependence. As Campbell (1984, p. 93) says, in a memorable statement:

> 'The power of medicine then becomes the power of letting go control, using knowledge of the limitations of medical work to encourage the patient to take part in the shared task of trying to understand and deal with the illness as it affects his or her personal being. [Thus] the doctor as God must be replaced by the fallible human being whose knowledge is incomplete and whose will is corruptible.'

We would argue that this 'identification with the other that lets go of self and self-importance' is the ultimate discipline of medical practice, provided it is a genuine outreaching and entry into the other person and their individual situation, and thus a true and authentic transcendence of one's self (see also Campbell, 1984, p. 77).

The therapeutic relationship of wise doctor and valued patient

This should not be confused, however, with setting aside professional knowledge and giving in to the patient's every whim, or responding unthinkingly to the needs and interests that the patient expresses. The patient's perception of what will help him/her is not always the best one. But it does mean that the knowledge of what is best for the patient is most likely to be gained through a meeting of the world of the patient and the doctor's world of professional knowledge and expertise. However, we should remember at the same time that 'a professional's knowledge of what constitutes goodness is really no better than anyone else's' (Campbell, 1984, p. 93).

To achieve this, the doctor has to tune in to the 'voice of the patient's body', and be the ally of body and/or psyche in helping a person restore a lost balance. He/she also has to learn to question his/her own assumptive world and help the patient grow beyond the assumptions on which help was first sought and offered. This is about responding to the 'rhythms, harmonies and balances of nature'. But it is more than this. It is also the 'effort to heal, to care for, or to support emotionally, which resists specification in precise tasks, and for which knowledge at an intellectual level is appropriate'. Yet there is something even beyond this, which Campbell sums up in the phrase 'the secular sacrament of medical care' (Campbell, 1984, pp. 96–100).

The consistent, respectful and valuing attention, which a humane doctor can offer a damaged fellow human being, draws upon a vision that sees – beyond the present starkness to the green shoots of hope and or faith – to something just beyond the periphery of our view. As Campbell (1984, p. 112) says:

> 'this can certainly become hubris, that vying with God to which medical practice is so prone, and it may lead to a heroic medicine which denies our mortality, but it need not be arrogance of this kind. A caring response to someone who may soon die creates and discovers the value which cannot be destroyed. It refuses to discard the person because the organism is decaying. This is the secular sacrament of medical care.'

This leads us to the non-rational in professional work, where help is given in mysterious ways (which Campbell calls 'the sacrament of the cup of cold water'), which links us back to the Picasso painting.

But care is not an act of giving, but an act of gratitude! Care provides for the carer a sense of fulfilment. It is easier to be a giver than a receiver. Care enables awareness of how much one gains in giving. As Campbell (1984, p. 107) reminds us:

> 'It is often more blessed to care than to be cared for; and the ability to care is frequently made possible by the understanding and sensitivity of the needy person. Such reciprocity suffuses the relationship of caring with a spontaneity, a sense of grace which enriches carer and cared-for alike.'

Patients feel cared for when their need is recognized and when the help that is offered does not overwhelm them but gently restores their strength at a pace that allows them to feel part of the movement to recovery. What makes them feel helpless and vulnerable is having a sense that they must conform to someone else's ideas of what they need.

Campbell (1984, p. 108) sums up the idea of 'being cared for rather than being managed', in the adjective 'graceful':

> 'Graceful care refers to something which is not offered by anxious people trying to earn love, but by sensitive people who release us from bonds of our own making in spontaneous and often surprising ways. The gracefulness in caring is as closely connected to bodily expression as it is to an intellectual understanding or emotional awareness.'

This brings us a new perspective on the doctor's power. The doctor may be invited to enter the doctor/patient relationship because of his/her knowledge and skill. This is the initial privilege that power accords. But, paradoxically, the therapeutic relationship will only be established and sustained by a very different form of knowing.

Knowing how you know what is best for the patient

Knowing what is best for anyone is a complex and elusive notion and we bring up to it both our individuality and our inevitably incomplete knowledge.

'The medieval synthesis of medicine and theology gave doctors a priest-like authority, since illness had always to be understood in relation to the healing of the sacraments and to the patient's eternal destiny' (Campbell, 1984, p. 25). Today, the scientific method apparently brings a different kind of power, thanks to which the position of the medical profession will probably always remain socially dominant. 'However modest and well-intentioned its practitioners, an aura of special influence tends to surround them. As a result there always remains the danger that "godlikeness" will obscure [their] ... limitations' (Campbell, 1984, p. 32).

This is nowhere more evident than in the danger that arises when the professional's assumptions about what is best for the client differ from the client's and the doctor–scientist wields the ultimate power and has the final say. Of course, medical power depends upon knowledge and skill, but it is a knowledge and skill that must itself be constantly altering to a wider and widening vision (see Chapter 10). Thus, as Campbell (1984, p. 26) states:

> 'the paternalistic claim to an unquestioned authority in health matters ... must be discarded if the true power of medicine is to be found. That power is found when the doctor genuinely listens to the patient and to the message of the illness and tries to transcend the limits of all previous understanding. It is the doctor as learner who carries a special authority, not the doctor as dogmatist.'

How far, then, is all this achievable by a professional who in the final analysis is merely a fallible human being?

The paradox of professionalism

It is in the light of all these perspectives on the invisible that Campbell (1984, pp. 82–3) argues that:

> 'the greatest problem for the professional helper is the demand for *agape* – the love which risks self in order to enhance value ... *Agape* requires that no help, however well intentioned, should stamp out one's own or another's individuality. Genuine help must see each person, including the helper, afresh, as a new and separate being, for whom no real parallel exists in prior experience – the unique encountering the unique.'

But he accepts that 'these requirements are more than can reasonably be expected', and returns to the paradox of professionalism in which the professional gains knowledge in order to help – but that knowledge gives both detachment and power, when what is needed instead is gracefulness and mutuality. Clearly, it is a hard demand to make on doctors that they should renounce the help that detachment offers in protecting themselves, and not use their knowledge and power for their own enhancement. (See Campbell (1984, pp. 83–4).) Clearly, this is about tipping the balance away from predominantly self-satisfying motives toward gratuitous concern for the welfare of others. It is important to remember that this is no more than the tipping of a delicate balance slightly to one side. It is not a plea to eliminate self-interest.

RESOURCES FOR LEARNING: A SERIES OF TRUE INSIGHTS

Resources 9.1–9.3 are to be used differently from those in previous chapters. They offer examples of true events relating to how patients see their doctors and what they remember of their interactions with them. These are designed to encourage doctors and their teachers to explore specifically what patients think about their care and how they see their doctors.

In particular, readers might ask: What qualities do patients look for in their doctors? Are they what you might expect?

In all three cases, the interaction between the doctor and the patient is at the core of the relationship. There is an over-simplistic idea that all that we have opened up here can be covered in communication skills courses. What is offered here is significantly more than communication skills, although what has been talked about are oral, physical and tacit aspects of communication. But we argue that 'communication' is not a simple, discrete skill. It has many forms, in some of which the tacit and sensory are more important than what is actually said.

If this is what can be said about the therapeutic relationship, to what extent is it paralleled in the relationship between the teacher and the learner?

Resource 9.1   Case One

The scene is a nightingale ward and it is 2.30 PM on a Friday afternoon. A 48-year-old male patient is being wheeled on a trolley out of the ward by two ambulancemen, on a journey that will take him home some 60 miles away. His family are waiting at home. Eight days before, he had an 'open-and-close' operation for inoperable oesophageal cancer. The ward doctor had jollied him along post-op and told him that he would improve more when he got home. As the trolley passes the doctor on the ward, the patient asks the ambulancemen to stop. He speaks gently and without malice and says 'You know Dr Jones, you should never lie to patients.' With that, the trolley is pushed out of the ward. The doctor is left with profound thoughts about this case, and finds that he is completely unprepared for how he was to be affected by this event. A period of thought and finally of written reflection leads to the following summary of the insights and resolutions of the ward doctor:

Insights

- I have to admit how silly I must have looked to the patient, who, despite no-one actually telling him, knew precisely what the score was: he was going home to die.
- I realize that I put my feelings (about wanting to offer the patient some encouragement and optimism) above the patient's, and therefore failed to gain an opportunity to have a meaningful conversation with this patient.
- This patient's case could not be cured, but I failed to offer him anything, because I did not admit that there was anything except cure.
- I failed to see the importance of healing as opposed to cure, and had missed a lot as a consequence.
- This patient's case can only help me if I use it to improve my practice.

Resolutions

- I vowed never to flinch from difficult discussions.
- I planned to run a teaching session with my colleagues, using this case as an example and using the heuristics to help their discussions.
- I vowed to read Chapter 3 of Kathryn Montgomery's book: 'Clinical judgement and the interpretation of the case' (Montgomery, 2006).

Resource 9.2   Case Two

It was a very hot August afternoon and the surgeon was at the local care home's annual fete. Halfway through the afternoon, the rather elegant elderly gentleman who had opened the fete approached and, touching his hat, said 'Elizabeth I must come and speak to you. You will probably not remember me but I was your patient seven years ago, Peter Williams ...' He offered his hand, in the gesture of a handshake. The surgeon returned the greeting and recalled that he had had a gangrenous gallbladder. 'Yes,' said the man, 'but you know the thing I remember with utmost clarity is you telling me that I was not going to die. I can see you now and hear those words. They were very comforting.' They continued to walk in the grounds and enjoy the afternoon talking about their relatives who lived at the home.

- The patient recalled what the surgeon had said.
- The surgeon recalled the operation performed.
- They enjoyed common ground at the event.
- The patient had been scared at the time of his admission, having been very ill.
- The patient had wanted to thank the surgeon and tell her that he remembered her words, which at the time were important.
- The surgeon could not recall the precise conversation, but did remember how ill he had been.
- The surgeon might have been flattered and buoyed up by the patient's comments.

Resource 9.3   Case Three[a]

A year after my child's diagnosis, five months after her treatment ended, I didn't care about scientific fact or epidemiological probability. I heard a surgeon long in practice tell me my daughter would not die of breast cancer, and all the studies and statistics, the questions and data that I used for months to dismiss attempts to placate me died in my mouth. I leaned back in the passenger seat. It wasn't politeness or (except maybe for a split second) deference to someone who was giving me a ride to meet her. Instead I was silenced by his assumption of a clinical responsibility. It was not certainty he offered but his best judgement and the grounds on which he based it. It felt as solid as certainty and somehow more valuable because certainty, I knew, was not to be found. The situated particularity of his clinical judgement and, especially, his openness about its limits was oddly enough what made him trustworthy. Ironist that he no doubt was, he was not asking me to believe the facts, but him. Besides, her treatment was over; it was time.

In the next moment, I began to believe him. Something hard and despairing in me settled, quieted, then let go. 'Thanks', I said provisionally, hearing it from a long way off – maybe just a little bit performatively. Then, unexpectedly, I saw that soon I would mean it with my whole heart.

[a]Montgomery (2006, pp. 206–7).

THE PEDAGOGIC RELATIONSHIP BETWEEN WISE TEACHER AND VALUED LEARNER

We demonstrated in de Cossart and Fish (2005) the parallels between medical and educational practice (Table 9.1). This table shows parallels between medical procedures and educational ones. The following explores the relationship that should exist beneath these visible activities.

The pedagogic relationship

This book is designed to offer learning resources for the clinical setting and also facilitative ways of teaching (see Chapter 3). It is therefore highly pertinent to point out the strong parallels between the role of the doctor with the patient and that of the teacher with the learner. This is the case in relation to the individual invisible elements of the relationship and for the holistic view, both of which have been discussed in earlier sections of this chapter.

Figure 9.3 is an adaptation of Figure 9.2 to express the relationship between the teacher and learner. It will be seen that all that we said of the invisibles in relation to the doctor and the patient are also the case for the teacher/learner relationship. We shall now explore this in more detail.

What is involved in the pedagogic relationship?

The relationship between learner and teacher is as privileged as that between doctor and patient. It is concerned with educational development, but at its heart is the drive to enable the learner to discover the fullest potential in themselves and to become independent from the teacher. It is not about a dependent relationship where the learner imitates or seeks to become like the teacher. At postgraduate level particularly, it is about developing a critique of both the theory the learner meets and the practice they engage in. It indicates the mutual *working together* of a wise teacher collaboratively with a learner. As we have already described above in relation to the patient/doctor collaboration, it requires a learner who is willing not merely to meet the teacher, but, where appropriate, to reveal to the teacher the particularity of their understanding and the individuality of their being. Here

Table 9.1 Parallels between medical and educational practice[a]

MEDICAL PRACTICE	EDUCATIONAL PRACTICE
Collaboration with patient – The doctor must:	**Collaborative with learner – Teacher and learner together must:**
1 Take history and examine	Find out what the learner knows and needs – during educational induction
2 Develop working diagnosis	Review learner's previous achievements and current needs in the light of what the attachment can offer
3 Carry out investigations	Explore current abilities in the clinical setting by review of educational portfolio
4 Review results and formulate treatment plan with patient	Agree learning intentions for the attachment and associated assessments and keep under regular review using formative assessment
5 Treat	Plan learning opportunities and agree what learner and teacher need to do, and carry this out
6 Review treatment	Review learning, through learner's reflective talking and writing
7 Treat complications	Plan for additional needs as they arise
8 Reconsider whole process	Learner to write a review of their achievements during the attachment
9 Record data and outcome (audit)	(a) Record summative assessment of learner's achievements in the attachment by reference to formative assessments (b) Record evaluation of the quality of the learning opportunities and the attachment as a whole
10 Discharge patient (requires medical knowledge, knowledge of Trust's systems, processes and record-keeping)	Sign-off learner (requires educational understanding of the learner and the nature of learning, knowledge of methods of supporting and assessing learning and methods of educational evaluation, and knowledge of the Trust and the Deanery's educational systems, processes and record-keeping)

[a] de Cossart and Fish (2005, p. 55).

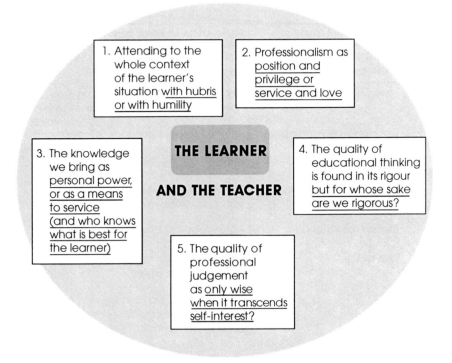

1. Attending to the whole context of the learner's situation with hubris or with humility

2. Professionalism as position and privilege or service and love

3. The knowledge we bring as personal power, or as a means to service (and who knows what is best for the learner)

THE LEARNER

AND THE TEACHER

4. The quality of educational thinking is found in its rigour but for whose sake are we rigorous?

5. The quality of professional judgement as only wise when it transcends self-interest?

Figure 9.3 The key elements at the core of education.

again, such a 'willingness' depends more on how the teacher meets the learner than on the character of the learner.

In order to achieve this, teachers have to pick their way through a number of educational complexities and ambiguities and lose the focus on themselves in order to 'study the learner'. Wisdom in working like this is not gained overnight. Neither is it without cost. But it does provide an ideal to aspire to (and sometimes to reach).

Such an approach to education involves the teacher in a commitment to each learner, which (though not limitless) certainly involves active concern, a will to work with rather than on the learner, and a kind of open-ended helpfulness (Campbell, 1984, p. 104). This, we believe, requires balancing a commitment to each learner with one to all other learners and (in medical education) to the best interests of patients. What we have said earlier about the practice of medicine is also true of the practice of education. It is about professing: service to mankind; disinterested love (a valuing of the other that takes full interest in them, without personal gain of any kind – including seeking a reputation for wisdom); and respect for every persons' dignity and rights (see p. 168).

As in medicine, in education this personal commitment cannot be captured solely in the current language of the 'contract'. It is a relationship that goes beyond 'codes of conduct' or guarantees of trustworthiness as safeguarded by professional codes of ethics and the disciplining of those whose conduct lies outside the acceptable.

At the heart of being a wise teacher are both the motivations and ethical principles that he/she brings as a professional educator and also the ability to recognize, navigate through and resolve (temporarily) the ambiguities inherent in 'serving another'. That is why most of the rest of what we have said above about the therapeutic relationship between doctor and patient (except the passage about bodily contact) applies equally in educational terms to the teacher/learner relationship.

END-NOTE

The day before the teaching seminar

Doctor to Foundation and Specialty programme doctors:

Tomorrow, we have a session to talk about the doctor/patient relationship (my term for communication skills, which I hate). I would like you all to spend some time tonight reading this letter that I received from a patient. From your own experiences and perhaps with the prompts of these resources [*hands over Resources 9.1–9.3*] bring a few written points that you have learned about the doctor/patient relationship from these cases.

The teaching seminar

The Doctor leads; there are about eight other doctors.

Doctor: OK who would like to start us off? …

David: Well I guess the patient had never felt listened to before this interview despite the fact that she obviously had been talked to … She says so in her letter. What specifically did you say to her to convince her that she was OK?

Doctor: I did not say anything new. She did most of the talking and I filled in several times on some points like the key elements of the treatment she had received, and why she had needed it, and made her tell me what she understood before she left.

Katy: But didn't that take a long time? Your clinic was running very late yesterday. Could someone else not have done it?

Doctor: Well she had been seen by several other doctors and healthcare professionals, but she seemed to be getting nowhere. I felt it was my responsibility to spend a little more time with her as after all I had been responsible for her cancer treatment. I had seen her before the treatment but actually this was my first meeting with her since she had gone home.

Katy: I suppose she trusted you and needed your advice.

Doctor: I think it was more than advice. She had been offered all that quite correctly before. It was her feeling that I needed to speak to her. She has had several life-changing events recently. Her husband was my patient three years ago and had a particularly unpleasant disease. He died last year. I think I gave her the chance to talk to the person that was at the centre of her cancer treatment. Time will tell what effect it has had.

James: Well it has obviously had the effect of making her write to you. That must be a start for her. She seems to have summarized things very well. How will you handle her next visit?

Doctor: Good question James. I have of course written to her family doctor and she will visit her before that visit. I will probably see her myself but she may need some extra time.

Six months later, the day after a clinic

Katy: Oh by the way, I saw Mrs Thomas in the clinic yesterday ... the lady we talked about in the seminar. She was down to see you, but you were running late and so the nurse brought her in to me. She sends her best wishes and said to say that she is sleeping much better and is about to go to Cornwall to visit her sister. There is no sign of cancer problems.

Doctor: Mmmmm good. Now are you going to match up what you have understood about this case with your previous notes? What better understanding do you have now of this case? Do you have something to tell your other colleagues about this case? Perhaps you should ...

FURTHER READING

Berger J, Mohr J (1967) *A Fortunate Man: The Story of A Country Doctor.* Harmondsworth: Penguin. [This is a very short read, but is but very moving, and is a classic in medical literature.]

Campbell A (1984) *Moderated Love: A Theology of Professional Care.* London: SPCK. [This book is very difficult to get hold of, but is well worth the effort. Two of its chapters are about nursing and social work, but most are about medicine. We know of no other publication of this kind and quality.]

Heath I (1995) *The Mystery of General Practice.* London: The Nuffield

Provincial Hospitals Trust. [This entire booklet is easy to read in a short space of time, and is very thought-provoking. It too is a classic.]

Neuberger J (2005) *The Moral State We're In: A Manifesto for a 21st Century Society.* London: HarperCollins. Introduction. [Much of this book goes beyond our subject here, but the introduction, brief though it is, is very valuable. Other chapters on the elderly and the mentally ill are also relevant.]

10

Seeing the clinical setting anew: Broadening the vision, deepening the insight

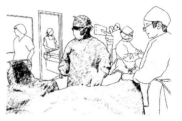

You are invited to keep the following in mind as you read this chapter:

Notes in preparation for writing an overview of my progress

1. What have I learned about myself so far?

- I had a rather fixed way of thinking ... 'thinking about how I think' has been very revealing ...
- I concentrated on the particulars of diagnosis and treatment before. They are important, but I didn't see my role in the wider context of the patient case.
- I need to get more succinct, logical and relevant in presentation. ... Especially when leading the care of the patient ... I need to be sure that I have thought through *and can defend* my decisions. Communication with staff, patients and relatives means I must expect to have formulated a plan and discussed it ... and if necessary reformulated it. I now see the importance of pulling together all the strands related to a patient case ...
- I must not let a patient and their relatives feel ignored ... it can be a significant source of resentment and frustration. I had assumed that juniors I left to do things would do them as I expected ... doesn't happen ... need to explain more. Same with hospital systems.
- I need to become more sceptical about things, and more critical. Being taken seriously has to be worked on ... doesn't come with the territory.

2. What can I do now that I could not before?

- Make and act on decisions based on my own and my consultant's assessment of my abilities.
- Conduct more effective – and even more efficient – ward rounds than before.
- Am developing new procedural skills that I did not have before.
- I anticipate better when things might go pear-shaped and pre-empt this outcome (not always – but better than before).
- I prioritize work better than I did.

3. What aspects of practice am I aware of now that I just took for granted before?

- My thinking processes (as above)
- Other people in the immediate environment of my practice (patients, managers, colleagues across the professions), but not sure exactly how their practice relates to mine (assuming it does!).

4. What do I now see out of the corner of my eye that I was not aware of before?

- Something about the greater complexity of practice ... and of all the people involved ... and something about how different people seem to bring different interpretations of a case ... and how to manage that.

5. What do I need to bring from the periphery of a patient case into the centre of my vision?

- I need to focus more on how systems work and what effect my decisions and actions will have on others ... especially the individual patient. Need to know more about other staff (nurses, OTs, physios, social workers) ... need to go out of my way to meet them ... see what they do and how it relates to what I do ...
- I need to bring teaching to the 'front burner'. I need to look at how I am taught in the clinical setting and to think about how to help others to learn in this environment.

6. How will I continue to develop these things?

- Make sure that I think, talk and write reflectively about cases, my practice, the wider things I am learning. ... Start actively finding out about colleagues' practice and managerial systems. ...

Some questions to consider as you read this chapter
- How has exploring the invisibles affected my everyday practice?
- How have they extended my awareness of the complex scene around me?

- What exactly do I now see in the clinical picture that I did not see previously?
- How has exploring the invisibles affected how I prepare to teach learners?
- What do I now need to work on further in respect of becoming an expert clinician?
- What are the implications of medicine being a social as well as a scientific practice?
- In terms of costs and availability, what do I see as the challenges to doctors in the 21st century and to healthcare more generally?

INTRODUCTION

Doctors have to attend to the development of their practice even while they are working as clinicians. Using the invisibles to explore practice can, we believe, contribute to doctors' development throughout their careers. Further, these elements that are the core of medicine, both singly and together, can provide a rigorous means to collect the evidence of achievement needed at all stages of career progression. This chapter focuses on how the invisibles can be used by maturing doctors to extend and chart further understanding and increasing wisdom.

In order to explore these matters fully, this chapter is divided into six sections. Firstly, we explore in more detail what is involved in becoming a wise practitioner. Secondly, we look at the invisibles' contribution to understanding and developing wise clinical practice as a holistic enterprise. Thirdly, we consider how to develop a discerning eye and how this is enhanced by the investigation of practice in order to refine it. Fourthly, we return to assessment and note how the processes we offer in this chapter can be used to prepare for assessment. Fifthly, we provide our final heuristic, which, in bringing us back to the complex clinical setting, reminds doctors that their focus needs to be widened and deepened to take in more and more of what is currently only in the periphery of their vision. Finally, we present three resources followed by some additional reading, to support doctors as they continue to explore further their daily practice and develop their wisdom.

BECOMING A WISE PRACTITIONER

The characteristics of a wise doctor: the goal to aim for

Medical practice is about particular cases and human events. A wise doctor draws together knowledge of and understanding about the complexity of clinical practice as a whole in order to provide the expert care and attention that each individual and different patient undoubtedly deserves. This requires a judicious balancing of the general and the particular, of science and art, and of fact and interpretation.

Developing the Wise Doctor

The wise doctor is a discerning doctor. The mark of an expert clinician is their ability to see more within every medical scenario than can their inexperienced colleagues. As they seek to become experts in patient care, new doctors will broaden and deepen their vision by developing a discerning eye about aspects of practice that are as yet only in the periphery of their view or that lie beneath the obvious aspects of the immediate case and their role in it.

A doctor with increasing expertise and maturity is also interested in the wider medical community. The mark of such a senior professional is their grasp of the significance of making a contribution to the professional development of their colleagues and the progress of their profession, at hospital level, Deanery level and national level. Such a contribution will be the more telling if it is founded both on a rigorous exploration of and ability to articulate the tacit and implicit in clinical practice, and also on a sound understanding of what makes for a wise doctor.

The wise doctor is one who brings the following to every particular medical event experienced:

- a recognition of the salient elements of the context and of the tradition within which they work
- an ability to articulate the relevant personal elements of the beliefs and assumptions that underlie their thought processes and actions
- an awareness of the significance of their professional values (both espoused values and values in use)
- a refined understanding of a wide range of the forms of knowledge they draw upon, together with an ability to select the salient, reject the irrelevant and generate practice knowledge
- an engagement in and the ability to be explicit about the rigour of their clinical thinking
- a facility in coming to wise judgements that they can defend articulately
- the ability to establish a sound therapeutic relationship with every patient, no matter how difficult or unappealing.

Becoming a wise doctor: the processes, stages and responsibilities

It is now generally recognized (across most professions) that in learning to become a good professional, 'practice' alone is not the all-encompassing activity it was once held to be. Of course, learning to practise involves gaining more and more experience. But having experiences without reflecting upon them rigorously is to waste some of their educational value and potentially to 'practise the wrong thing, or practise in the wrong way'. The role of reflection in learning to practise is – quite simply – essential. It is how to derive meaning from what would otherwise be a procession of discrete and partly understood events. It is a means of making more of every experiential opportunity, and can compensate in part for the shorter postgraduate period now available for learning to be a doctor.

Resource-based learning, we have argued, provides less experienced doctors with a means of developing senior expertise. As an educational method, it is sound, and as a means of learning to develop and refine clinical practice, it is apt and appropriate. Using resources to explore their own practice and their understanding of that practice provides doctors with a means of investigating their practice. It will ultimately drive the curriculum model behind the education of doctors from the process model to the research model (see above: pp. 44–49).

We believe that learning to become a wise doctor involves a cyclical process. This cycle may begin with the inexperienced doctor developing an awareness of the implicit and tacit elements that drive visible performance. This may be followed by a first exploration of each invisible and how present practice may be understood in the light of them. This should lead on to the critique of theory in the light of practice (both theory about the invisibles and about the learning resources offered) and practice in the light of theory (both the doctor's own practice and practice more generally).

But the learning process will only come to full maturity when all these individual elements come holistically together to inform, enlighten and refine clinical practice through reflection-in-action (during practice) and reflection-on-action (before and after practice). When this happens, both at the patient's 'bedside' and 'beyond' (during the daily cut and thrust of busy and bustling human interaction and medical complexity), the doctor will begin to see anew both their own practice and clinical practice generally. They will reflect more often and more deeply and provide increasingly richer narratives of their practice. They will also see that practice in a context far wider than their local hospital Trust environment. They will then want to investigate their practice and its clinical context, and push out further the boundaries of their understanding of it. Thus they will begin to drive their own learning and develop greater discernment.

But even this will not be the end. What Gawande says of learning to be a surgeon is true for all doctors. It involves an endless 'recapitulation of the process – the floundering, followed by the fragments, followed by knowledge and occasionally a moment of elegance – over and over again, for even harder tasks with ever greater risks' (Gawande, 2001, p.22). And as the tasks become harder, the invisibles begin to reveal new levels of complexity. This is why, when faced with these rising demands, the wise doctor may find it useful to return to the beginning of this cycle of learning about the invisible elements of practice. This time, the doctor may use them (or some of them) individually, to sharpen understanding of the new demands of practice, and call on them together in order to develop a renewed vision of the holistic nature of their professional role as medical practitioners.

In achieving this, they will be drawn to investigate their activities as doctors and thus arrive at the real nub of personal professional development.

DEVELOPING WISE, HOLISTIC PRACTICE IN THE CLINICAL SETTING

This section takes a new look at the invisibles and offers ways of extending the six invisible elements so far offered into a seventh that brings them all together and provides ways of developing wisdom throughout a doctor's postgraduate career.

Firstly, we return to basic principles by asking a deeper question about medical practice than we have tackled before. That question is: What is 'a practice'? Then, in order to consider how we learn a practice, each of the invisibles in turn is examined for how they contribute to a professional's increasing maturity of practice.

What is a practice?

A 'practice' is a term for any more or less settled body of activities that is carried out to some distinctive end. Here, 'activities' means particular things people do to some overall social purpose. Golby and Parrott (1999) offer parenthood as an example, and we draw on their ideas in what follows.

In parenting, for example, particular activities have a regular place that may be more or less settled or agreed. Examples would be bedtime routines, methods of discipline, family holidays and excursions, and visits to grandparents. When all the activities that generally characterize this 'practice of parenthood' are taken together, they provide a way of understanding individual parents' practice of parenting, the means of talking about any individual versions of parenting as, for example, 'loving' or 'cold', 'permissive' or 'highly disciplined'. Here, as Golby and Parrott point out, evidence for such descriptions would come from examples of particular activities pursued by the parents in question.

However, they note that making generalizations from the particular is more difficult. For example, what counts as a characteristic activity and what is seen as its value to the entirety of 'that practice' are potentially contentious and controversial issues about which conventional wisdom changes over time. For example, the Victorian *paterfamilias* is no longer a popular figure. Further, each and every family has its own decisions to make about such issues, whether explicitly and deliberatively or by default through habit. Thus, it is not in direct generalizing from the particular that a national practice comes to be established. As Golby and Parrott (1999, p. 13) say: 'In establishing the character of your own practice of parenthood you are at the same time contributing to the general practice, though in what may seem a small way. Nevertheless, a contribution it is, and one that makes itself felt most in the subsequent influence it has on your grown up children and their own practice of parenthood.' In a sense, then, you are building a tradition.

Learning to work within a tradition of practice

Learning to be a doctor, like learning to be a parent, is learning to work within the traditions of practice and learning to contribute to them. This does not mean that doctors as they learn the practice of medicine should be *confined* within those traditions. Indeed, critique and development of ideas and activities must be part of any profession's traditions. But it does mean that the traditions in which they are brought up will shape how doctors see, think and act. This will be true for all but the utterly brilliant doctor who by inventing original ways of working will cause a seismic shift in the traditions of a practice and thereby take practice into a new realm. This has serious educational implications, and indicates the size of the responsibility that teachers in professional practice have for learners (even when such teachers are only incidental models of practice for a doctor who is passing by).

How then is a practice learnt? Over time, practitioners develop the following: ways of seeing the world; ways of doing things; ways of regarding issues and problems; and ways of talking about matters of practice. In supporting professionals as they learn 'a practice', teachers need to ensure that the embedded or implicit aspects of practice are made overt. This brings with it key responsibilities.

Learning to 'do medicine' is inextricably bound up with learning to 'be a doctor', learning to 'think like a doctor' and learning to 'see in the way that doctors see'. Thus, maturing in medical practice is far from just acquiring or developing new skills and theoretical knowledge and using them more or less as one pleases as a lone expert. As Golby and Parrott (1999, p. 13) say:

'The skills and techniques of a practice are not neutral instruments to be used to satisfy whatever desires a particular individual may happen to have. The way we see the world, what we try to achieve in it and how we go about trying to do so are not independent of one another. We see and behave as we do primarily because we act in accordance with a way of seeing and doing laid down by a tradition and because people who belong to that tradition see and behave in that way.'

How then can we characterize the practice of medicine in respect of these matters? What will maturing doctors need to come to grips with?

Practice: the context for doctors' professional development

Medicine is a social as well as a scientific practice. For doctors, this provides a very significant context for learning to practice.

For example, doctors work in the centre of a world in which the laws of science are in sharp conflict with the colloquial wisdom of lived practice (Montgomery, 2006, p. 104). In all their decisions and actions, they have to be able to keep the balance successfully between medicine as a science and medicine as an art; between medicine as a scientific practice and medicine as a social practice; between honouring their particular profession's traditions of conduct and recognizing that they are not the sole agents and arbitrators of health provision (and that other professions have their different traditions).

But it is even more complex than this. Doctors have to live in a world where there are many wrong 'answers' and no right ones. They have to balance the colloquial, human and humane wisdom about practice that emanates from the social world of medicine (and which itself is full of contradicting aphorisms that offer no reliable way forward), with the rigid, definitive and absolute wisdom of science, which is no more helpful, being full of invariant laws that do not reflect real life and that also fail to provide right answers for individuals.

All this means that doctors have to negotiate successfully with a wide range of people in the clinical setting. And this requires the personal commitment, motivation and vision to attend to all this, as well as awareness of the beliefs and assumptions that colour the lens through which they look and the sense that they make of the world. This is no easy and soft option, neither is it an insignificant element in becoming a successful doctor. Getting this wrong can lead to the label 'dysfunctional doctor' and cause grief to both patients and colleagues. In developing professional practice, context is everything.

What complicates this further is that contexts are dynamic in their very nature. The circumstances of a patient case and the context in which a doctor responds to it (and all other aspects of the practice of medicine) are liable to frequent change. This will affect how, when and why the doctor uses and creates knowledge, as well as affecting the doctor's own frame of reference (his/her needs, values, beliefs and assumptions). Thus, as and when appropriate, the doctor will have to reconsider matters of context and of personal qualities and capacities. It is of course a professional judgement as to when this is appropriate, when to remain adamant about matters and when to be flexible.

In other words, the practice context in which doctors learn medicine is itself uncertain and ambiguous, and this affects the understanding and use of all the invisibles, as follows.

Clinical thinking in the complex practice setting

What Montgomery (2006, p. 103) says of new doctors emerging from medical school in America is probably true of UK graduates: ' ... luckily they are intelligent, but they are also (most of them) longtime [sic] students of science who are not used to negotiating ambiguous alternatives or to tolerating incomplete or uncertain answers'. How then should doctors proceed in learning the wisdom in clinical thinking that is so central to the practice of medicine?

There is no simple easy answer. Learning 'a practice' has to be worked at *in practice*. For example, doctors need to look more carefully at what is involved in the lived experience of coming to a professional judgement. They need to recognize what actually makes it complex, and they need to find ways of coping with this. This will include keeping a judicious balance between competing ways of seeing and thinking, maintaining a scepticism about 'solutions', and engaging personal professional judgement throughout the Clinical Thinking Pathway. These all need to be practised and reflected upon more and more richly and more and more honestly.

We have already seen that becoming a wise doctor is partly a matter of engaging in clinical thinking in terms of both the scientific 'clinical reasoning' and the 'humanistic' deliberation. But if they look carefully, doctors trying to use this in the clinical setting will also come to recognize that they are pressed to draw on competing forms of 'wisdom'. At crucial moments, they are often offered by their seniors 'conventional wisdom'. This is captured in aphorisms (witty, common sayings) – many of which contradict each other. (A medical example would be 'always trust the patient', but at the same time 'never believe that the patient knows everything'!) How then should the doctor proceed?

As Montgomery (2006, p. 111) puts it: 'medicine's paired and counterweighted aphoristic wisdom' feeds into all aspects of practical reasoning, challenging the science and introducing ever more ambiguity. For example, even in history-taking, medical tradition has it both that the patient will, if properly attended to, tell you the diagnosis, but also that the patient is a very unreliable historian. This ambiguity affects the physical examination also, where traditional 'wisdom' says both 'fit your clinical observations to known patterns' and the opposite: 'take account of every detail and weigh them carefully'. Everywhere there are ill-fitting elements, and problems about whether to 'go along with' those details that are immediately apparent or with the wider pattern of signs and symptoms. See Montgomery (2006, Chapter 7) for an extremely useful detailed exploration of this.

Despite these difficulties, we would still advocate using the Clinical Thinking Pathway (its language and ideas) both to continue to explore these subtleties and perhaps also to use it to think through Trust-wide issues (see de Cossart and Fish, 2005, pp. 162–4), and more deeply personal ones, including, perhaps, in career planning and preparation for or reflection on RITA assessments or job interviews (see the later sections below). In all these activities, reaching wise judgement is the goal, and the pathway can help.

Exercising professional judgement in the complex practice setting

In addition to what we have said above, there are additional practice activities that require the exercise of professional judgement. These include issues such as the assessment of doctors' performance, understanding and progress (where there is no exact science, and never will be); how to develop a therapeutic relationship with all patients (even the less graceful, the more demanding and the positively uncongenial ones); and even the best way to investigate one's own practice in the complex clinical setting in a way that is rigorous but on an appropriately *small* scale (unlike scientific research, which is large-scale).

Using knowledge in the complex practice setting

We have already seen that the practice setting is a vital arena for the construction of new knowledge by practitioners themselves. Many healthcare professions are already familiar with this idea. Higgs *et al.* (2007), in the third edition of an already classic text on clinical reasoning for the healthcare professions, remind us that:

'professional judgement is utilized by practitioners in the selection of knowledge to be used *and* the kind of use to which that knowledge is put in the practice setting. Here, practitioners consider what is appropriate knowledge, how it might be used, and whether it should be modified to suit the particular case. That modification is itself a version of creating knowledge *in* practice.'

191

Developing the Wise Doctor

Doctors who wish to develop wise practice will need to look at, as well as talk and write in depth about, the knowledge they generate within their practice. In addition to considering the range of forms of knowledge that illuminate a particular patient case, they might also begin to recognize that knowledge is a social, historical and political construct, and begin to penetrate the implications of this for judgements about what are 'facts' and what are 'interpretations of facts'. Yesterday's facts may become today's myths!

Establishing good patient relationships at the same time as developing a wider awareness of the practice setting

Finally, in reviewing and seeing anew the invisibles in the practice setting, we are anxious to point out that although in Chapter 9 we emphasized the importance of focusing on the patient in order to establish a sound medical and therapeutic relationship with them, we also believe that such a focus should not be to the exclusion of developing an ever-sharper awareness of the entire clinical setting, where the patient and doctor are but part of the scene.

Indeed, just below the surface of much of what we have been saying is the idea that developing wise practice is centrally about developing a more discerning eye.

DEVELOPING 'THE DISCERNING EYE' – AND BECOMING AN INVESTIGATOR OF ONE'S PRACTICE

The act of noticing is itself important. As Higgs *et al.* (2007) say, 'Health care practitioners are expected to notice things; to become aware of their patients' needs and responses. They are expected to appraise critically their own performance, role and actions. In so doing they can become aware of patterns of behaviour and outcomes in their clinical interventions.' Looking more deeply and wider often leads to a realization that there is ever more to attend to at the periphery of one's vision and thus the periphery of one's practice.

Doctors who are relatively new to medical practice focus almost exclusively on the immediate circle of their own activities (and those of their clinical supervisor). They are not even aware of what occurs at what would be the periphery of their vision. Thus learning to practise with greater maturity is about becoming aware of the wider view and drawing it more into focus. In order to 'see' as their expert senior colleagues see, doctors must learn the habit of looking with 'a discerning eye' (Fish, 1998).

Developing the discerning eye

The doctor's discerning eye needs to take in the visible and see through to the invisible. The looking involved needs, for example, to be at the physical elements of practice (seeing the context in more detail and any need to investigate it further), at the more obscure elements of what one brings personally to practice, at the implications of being a professional, at the deeper meaning of the new knowledge one has generated in practice, at the range of subtle pressures on one's clinical thinking and action, at the longer-term outcomes of one's professional judgements, and at the costs of establishing a therapeutic relationship.

Such an 'appreciation' of the complexity of practice (when carried out by practitioners on their own practice and when conducted rigorously within the procedures of humanistic investigation) is seen in the heathcare professions generally as a form of practitioner research.

For doctors who believe that the only form of research is scientific research and the only reputable version of this is double-blinded randomized controlled trials, the following will be difficult. For those who recognize that the humanities and the social sciences have their own forms of research, it will be more congenial.

Going beyond reflection and appreciation: becoming a conscious investigator of one's own practice

Investigating one's practice in order to understand it better is an inevitable extension of reflecting on that practice and 'appreciating' it. The focus of such scrutiny is either on the gap that has been identified between one's ideals and intentions for practice and one's actual achievements, or it is on the wider context of one's practice when growing awareness alerts one to elements that have barely been glimpsed before. The ends to which these investigations are bent are those of improving the understanding of one's own practice in order to improve that practice itself, such that patients are better served, colleagues' roles are more fully acknowledged, and one's profession is thereby enhanced. This includes the ability to offer 'an account' of one's practice and thus to provide the basis for one's accountability.

The investigation of their practice by health care professionals (the principles of which are equally relevant to doctors) has been the topic of many major books, and readers are referred to these for a full exposition of the main research paradigms (world views) and the methods they involve. Examples of small investigations useful for doctors in the practice setting are contained in the resources below.

Trying to understand practice better is difficult, may be uncomfortable, can take time and is better worked on in respect of one small piece of practice rather than attempting a large-scale exploration. It involves both looking at difficult matters and finding words that express them adequately.

Yet in starting with a small but well-chosen piece of their own practice, professionals can quickly unravel some of the issues at its core and come to see them as relating to the heart of the profession's practice. The starting point for such enquiry, then, is intimate and highly detailed but it relates to wider issues and may ultimately be for a more public professional audience.

ASSESSMENT AS THE COLLECTION AND USE OF EVIDENCE OF MATURATION AND DEVELOPING WISDOM

Arguably the most important contribution of MMC to postgraduate medical education is to be found in its flagging-up of the need to collect evidence in and from the clinical setting as a means to assessing the achievements and progress of doctors and as the basis for decisions about their appointment and promotion.

Our arguments are that such evidence needs to be richer and more discriminating than is permitted by the tick-box forms used in 'Tools of the Trade'. However, the evidence documented by the C-bD and DOPS forms can be enriched by reflective accounts of the kind we have been promoting in the earlier chapters of this book. Even this approach to collecting evidence of maturation will not, however, be sufficient as the doctor proceeds further in his/her career. That is why we are advocating in this chapter the need for doctors themselves to collect a yet wider range of evidence about the invisibles within their own practice. The focus of such investigation is personal practice, but it will of course inevitably draw upon the views and understandings of others with whom the doctor works.

The starting point for such extended collection of evidence (and thus the assessment of the doctor) might well arise out of a reflective account of a case or a procedure, or might arise from some other event or incident in practice. Such a starting point (sometimes called a 'critical incident') will trigger some empirical investigation, some reading and thinking, and will result in a reflection on practice that links individual practice and what has been learnt about it, with wider professional ideas. However, where the starting point is a clinical event (or 'critical incident'), this should be carefully differentiated from an adverse incident, which must be considered by all clinicians involved in it for risk-management purposes.

Critical incidents as a starting point for investigation and written reflection

An adverse incident has to be reviewed in order to check the safety of systems and management of risk for patients' well-being. Here the focus is on the medical case and the events that surrounded it as well as the procedures and routines, protocols and guidelines that the Trust or Specialist bodies require doctors to use. That is, an adverse incident has a medical focus and is about medical processes.

Exploring a clinical event for educational purposes (which includes accruing the evidence used for assessing the doctor) is quite different. Here, the focus is on the *doctor*. Here, the incident is 'critical' in that it has significance for the doctor as a learner. The incident can be a very ordinary happening that is imbued with importance by the doctor, for whom it raises a question or poses a value conflict.

Using critical incidents educationally rests on the understanding that learning is a response to both experience and personal interest in that experience. In order to move beyond our 'everyday, working way of looking at things' we need to 'arrest' (i.e. freeze the frame of) a significant moment in our experience in a way that renders it open to analysis and critique. We then need to see such moments – and ourselves – anew. We need to 'render the familiar strange' and thus to see our ideas, beliefs, assumptions, and theories from a different perspective.

Table 10.1 offers a summary of the contributions that can be made to the assessment of a doctor by three means: 'Tools of the Trade'; the use of the invisibles; and the processes of investigation of practice by the practitioner (usually referred to as 'practitioner research'). It will be seen from this table that both the invisibles and practitioner research make a useful contribution to evidence for assessment. The issue of the part played by standards in assessment is pursued in the appendix following this chapter. In considering how the invisibles enrich the assessment and the standards in medicine, it offers a table that summarizes the key elements of a doctor's clinical practice that arguably should be assessed if the nature of that practice is to be properly attended to. For each element, it demonstrates the difference in charting standards between 'Tools of the Trade' on the one hand and the invisibles (now including this final invisible of 'seeing beyond') on the other. Identifying the aspects of postgraduate medicine to be assessed and pinpointing the assessment methods is a way of identifying the areas of the curriculum that postgraduate doctors will take seriously. The appendix therefore provides an overview of how we are seeking to enrich the current curriculum.

HEURISTIC 7: BROADENING THE VISION, DEEPENING THE INSIGHT

Heuristic 7 (Figure 10.1) attempts to capture all that we have said about doctors developing a discerning eye and needing to be aware of and to investigate further

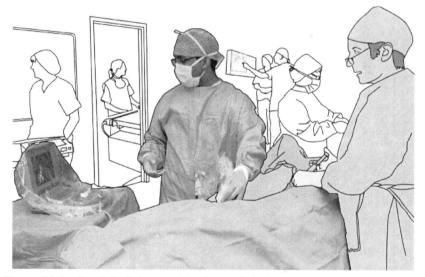

Figure 10.1   Heuristic 7: beyond the immediate focus.

Table 10.1 A summary of three different kinds of assessment methods and the evidence they generate

	'Tools of the trade'	Reflective narratives based on the resources for exploring 'the invisibles'	Practitioner research
Resources	The resources are the forms designed to be optically read	The resources are narratives of practice, designed to support the exploration of 'the invisibles' of practice	The resources are the processes of action research, case study or conversation analysis
Who does it?	A wide range of assessors, but with little continuity (different on each occasion)	This is done by the learner and checked by the clinical supervisor and/or educational supervisor (there is continuity here)	This is done by the learner and checked by the clinical supervisor and/or educational supervisor (there is continuity here)
Process of documentation	Some aspects of the visible elements of practice are documented in the heat of practice	Reflection on action unearths the invisible elements of practice from a rich range of perspectives, which are documented outside practice	This allows practitioners themselves to explore further, inside and outside practice, elements they have identified for further attention, and deepening understanding
Quality of evidence	Mainly tick-box evidence of achievement on a given date, whose meaning (and standards) may be unclear to later supervisors	Written reflection and the chance to offer a summary across narratives and thus to chart developing insight that is easily understood and reviewed by subsequent supervisors	A reflective report that presents what was investigated, how and what has been learnt by the learner about own practice. It thus exposes the quality of the learner's thinking and understanding of own practice and how it relates to others' practice and understanding. This provides evidence easily reviewed by subsequent supervisors

those elements of practice that are at the periphery of their vision. This we have characterized as 'going beyond' both what individual invisibles can offer and what the doctor has achieved in the earlier stages of practice.

THE RESOURCES

Resource 10.1: Investigating practice

The basic means that doctors can use to collect evidence to fuel consideration of their own practice are captured in Resource 10.1, which combines traditional methods of collecting data with some new ways of using the invisibles and the resources associated with them. It should be noted that 'investigation' in this sense is not an activity designed to 'investigate and inspect colleagues and systems', and it is not to be used in order to set them right, but to gain information that will enrich the doctor's own understanding of his or her own practice and its context.

Resource 10.1   Some useful methods of collecting evidence in practitioner research

Focus of investigation	Method	Means of collecting evidence
• More of what is involved in the complexity of the practice setting (events associated with a ward round and clinic management)	• Observation	• Own observation • Observation of others • Written notes/ tables/maps
• Own abilities in talking to/with colleagues, patients and learners (any practice setting)	• Collection of spoken conversation	• Tape recording, transcription and analysis
• How the hospital system is managed	• Interviews with managers/ administrators/ colleagues/patients • Mapping relationships	• Semistructured interview (same key questions to everyone) plus emerging category analysis (seeing what patterns and categories emerge)

Focus of investigation	Method	Means of collecting evidence
		• Mind maps – any means of turning information into diagrams (and checking these back with interviewees)
• How one manages a case	• Reflection • Interviewing colleagues, patients, administrators	• Own reflective writing (do this first); semi-structured interviews; correlate emerging issues with own understanding as shown in writing
• How seniors come to professional judgements • MDT meeting	• Observation of and questions to individuals • Use of the Invisibles in an MDT meeting	• Own observation and key questions • Use the clinical thinking pathway and the professional judgement chart to trace the arguments when complex cases are discussed by senior clinicians in MDT meetings
• Self as a learning doctor	• Case study	• Use reflection and interviews to study the patient case and self as a learning doctor

Resource 10.2: Some sources of conflicting values that make demands on clinical practice

Professionals have to find ways on the spot of resolving conflicts, in specific instances of practice, and between differing publicly required values that they find to be at odds with each other and their own. These are eternally 'problematic' and have to be wrestled with in every patient case, because there is never a once-for-all resolution which will fit every case. Knowing what you wish to prioritize can help.

Resource 10.2 offers a sharp reminder of these conflicting values that exert pressure on the professional doctor's daily work, and the sources from which they come. This resource can be useful when exploring and seeking to resolve problems arising from conflict within a team about what to do and why and how to do it.

It illustrates the variety of people and places whose values come to bear on the practice of medicine in the secondary sector of the NHS. The varied shapes indicate differences in ways of prioritizing values and differences in the amount of pressure of these on the doctor's own professional life. At different times in the doctor's career the priority of the various influences will change, but they will always all be present.

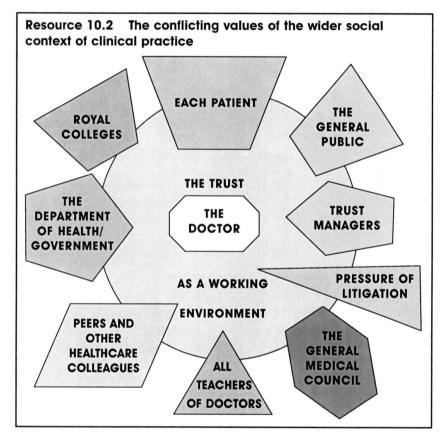

Resource 10.2   The conflicting values of the wider social context of clinical practice

ROYAL COLLEGES

EACH PATIENT

THE GENERAL PUBLIC

THE DEPARTMENT OF HEALTH/ GOVERNMENT

THE TRUST

THE DOCTOR

TRUST MANAGERS

AS A WORKING ENVIRONMENT

PRESSURE OF LITIGATION

PEERS AND OTHER HEALTHCARE COLLEAGUES

ALL TEACHERS OF DOCTORS

THE GENERAL MEDICAL COUNCIL

Readers might use this resource to help them to consider the sources of conflict in a team, or even within their own practice. They might also use it to explore the values of the individuals that make up the multiprofessional teams they work in, and to raise issues about the values of their professions.

Resource 10.3: Preparing yourself for assessment as the case of a learning doctor

We offer in Resource 10.3 an outline example of how the Clinical Thinking Pathway might be used by a maturing doctor (who is perhaps already beyond the

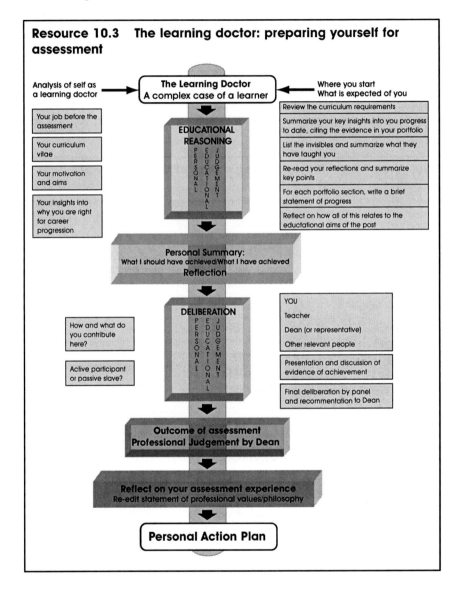

Resource 10.3 The learning doctor: preparing yourself for assessment

Foundation programme) as a means of preparing for a RITA assessment or an interview for a new post.

The end-of-chapter scenario that now follows builds upon the notes at the start of the chapter and uses the content of the chapter to put together a statement for the RITA panel that highlights educational achievement. It should be noted that this is not offered as an ideal example, but rather a typical one, which shows some weaknesses (for example, there is nothing about teaching in any detail here).

Personal statement for the RITA highlighting educational achievements

I have learned that I had a very fixed way of thinking, homing in on the complexity of the clinical case and the theoretical knowledge about treatment, and often missing the subtleties of the patient's opinion and thinking. I had a somewhat autocratic style of running a ward round, which involved me doing most of the talking. I am working on changing this and giving more room to my juniors to talk and think aloud so that I know better what they understand and what they don't. My investigations of this so far are to be found in Section 5 of the portfolio.

With respect to consultants and what they expected of me, I have realized that succinct, logical and relevant presentations are essential and that my rather didactic style was too long-winded (and actually able to be done by the nurse). I need to concentrate on making sound professional judgements about achievable patient care and checking them out with my seniors. I had been used to the consultant making all of these important decisions, and I was just a follower. I am getting better at this and getting to be familiar with all the people and systems that invest in the care of the patient. I have been used to assuming that all those things automatically happened and had wondered on several occasions why things that I thought were clear had not been done.

I need to be more sceptical in my approach and not rely completely on the systems (especially since they are more and more driven by protocols, which sometimes I need to consider over-riding). I am getting better at prioritizing work and refining my decision-making and judgement so that I can defend them from any angle. I plan to get a better handle on those systems by finding out how the Trust policies on arrangements for elective and emergency admission actually work in practice.

I had laid much store on those junior to me having understood what I wanted (without actually checking it through with them). I have made a recording of myself explaining to juniors a particular aspect of a patient case that I wanted them to be involved with. The transcript of this has provided some points to work on. I think I am improving on that score. I had thought that they were getting involved with the patient and their relatives – but actually they were not proactive at all, and we have been addressing that in some of our tutorials.

I think my theoretical knowledge has improved and I am beginning to develop a discipline in checking up-to-date knowledge and evidence about cases. The IT access is useful for this, but on ward rounds we now regularly discuss how much of the information offered

> should be used and when. I have been surprised how infrequently we follow to the letter the ideas in the published literature.
>
> I have been going out of my way to talk with specialist nurses, OTs, physios and social workers – much more than I had seen it necessary to do before – and I have seen the care and management of patients improve as a result.
>
> I have set up a group reflective writing session, which involves the nurses and the doctors, and I hope to continue this, as well as writing for my own use. I have been surprised how well received it has been and that it does not take huge lengths of time. (See Section 5b of my portfolio.)

We have sought throughout this book to show doctors what they can achieve when their education is based upon a more enriched curriculum than is currently available nationally. We believe that what we offer here can make a difference. We hope it will – but that is in the hands of readers.

FURTHER READING

Higgs J, Fish D, Rothwell R (2007) Knowledge generation and clinical reasoning in practice. In: Higgs J, Jones M, Loftus S, Christensen N, eds. *Clinical Reasoning in the Health Professions*, 3rd edn. Edinburgh: Elsevier.

Montgomery K (2006) *How Doctors Think: Clinical Judgement and the Practice of Medicine*. Oxford: Oxford University Press. [See especially Chapter 7.]

Appendix

Enriching the postgraduate medical curriculum

A summary of elements of clinical practice that can be developed and recorded, the standards that might be aimed for and an indication of how well the current assessment processes enable doctors to explore and document this, compared with what can be achieved if the invisibles' are also used.

Element of practice to be learnt and assessed, and standard to be aimed for	Assessment methods found in national curricula (mainly 'Tools of the Trade') and the quality of evidence they produce	Means of gaining evidence of the invisible aspects of practice and how the quality of evidence available relates to the standard to be achieved
1a. Practitioner's appreciation of the significance of context		
(i) Definition Understanding the effects on one's practice of the specific context of the case and the environment in which one first became responsible for the case	There is no means of assessing this, except indirectly through C-bD	**CONTEXTUAL ANALYSIS GUIDE (see p. 72)** **Note and reflect on all the relevant elements of the context that can affect practice: the clinician, colleagues, the patient, the immediate physical environment and the wider environment**
(ii) Standard to be achieved *The recognition of and ability to chart/record/pinpoint the salient points of the context for each patient case and for any other aspect of practice.*	All evidence collected in this way is superficial and does not relate to the standard	*In respect of the standard to be achieved, this offers a way of creating evidence of the subtleties and interpretative aspects of a situation and allows for reconsideration and development of these. It therefore provides clear evidence of whether the doctor has reached the standard and provides the basis for clarifying any remedial work necessary*

1b. Practitioner's personal qualities (as contributing to the context of clinical practice)

(i) Definition **The beliefs, assumptions, attitudes and values one demonstrates within one's practice and how they can affect it** **The demonstration of sensitivity, imagination and high interpersonal skills**	**Mini-PAT collects some evidence of how others see the doctor** (Never gets down to the level of values)	**THE ICEBERG OF PRACTICE** **(see p. 74)** **Use the iceberg of practice as a reminder of what the individual doctor, uniquely, brings to their practice**
(ii) Standard *The ability to articulate one's beliefs, assumptions, attitudes and values and how they affect one's practice; critique them; and set them on one side if they adversely affect the quality of patient care.* *To be a person who brings up to practice a wise and holistic humanity*	The evidence collected is indirect and incomplete and does not allow assessment with respect to the standard	*In respect of the standard to be achieved, this offers a rigorous way of identifying, exploring and developing these implicit/tacit elements of practice.* It therefore provides clear evidence of whether the doctor has reached the standard and provides the basis for clarifying any remedial work necessary

2. Practitioner's professional values

(i) Definition **One's professional values (both espoused values and values-in-action).** **Understanding how these affect the context of, the community of, the patients involved in, and one's actions within each case/practice**	There is no means of assessing this	Reflect on ideas offered in: **THE TABLE OF THE EXTENDED AND RESTRICTED PROFESSIONAL** **(see p. 86)** **MEMBERSHIP OF A PROFESSION** **(see p. 90)** **Begin to establish a statement of your professional philosophy**

Element of practice to be learnt and assessed, and standard to be aimed for	Assessment methods found in national curricula (mainly 'Tools of the Trade') and the quality of evidence they produce	Means of gaining evidence of the invisible aspects of practice and how the quality of evidence available relates to the standard to be achieved
2. Practitioner's [professional values *(contd.)*		
(ii) Standard *To be an extended professional, with full characteristics and values of a member of a profession*	There is no evidence to assess against the standard	*In respect of the standard to be achieved,* this offers a way of creating evidence of a rigorous consideration of the impact a practitioner can have on a clinical situation and the level of awareness the doctor has about his/her own professional qualities. It therefore enables clear evidence to be provided of whether the doctor has reached the standard and provides the basis for clarifying any remedial work necessary
3a. The forms of knowledge that the practitioner uses in practice		
(i) Definition **The ability to call upon a wide range of forms of knowledge in response to clinical practice and to draw upon the salient elements of all forms as appropriate**	**CASE-BASED DISCUSSION** **EXAMINATIONS** (mainly of propositional/ theoretical knowledge)	**THE KNOWLEDGE CARDS** **(see p. 110)** Use these to prompt you to consider the full range of knowledge you have drawn on in your practice

(ii) Standard *To have an ability to draw widely on forms of knowledge as appropriate to the particular practice; to be able to articulate these; to be able to organize the mind to make relevant knowledge quickly available in the practice setting; and to be able to critique the relevance of knowledge used in practice*	C-bD concentrates only on knowledge of the disease. Examinations assess only the possession of theoretical and factual knowledge Neither explores how knowledge is used in practice	*In respect of the standard to be achieved,* this offers practice in identifying and articulating the salient knowledge needed for a given case, and ways of developing a speedy codification of all that is needed in the case. It therefore enables clear evidence to be provided of whether the doctor has reached the standard and makes clear the basis for deciding the nature of any remedial work necessary

3b. Technical processes and procedures carried out by the practitioner (focus on procedural knowledge)

(i) Definition **The ability to carry out satisfactorily all key procedures required within clinical practice including technical and operative competence as appropriate to the specialty**	**DOPS and MiniCEX** **Triggered Assessment (TA)/Operative Competence (OP COMP), and Orthopaedic Curriculum Assessment Project (OCAPs) [in the surgical specialty curricula]**	**THE KNOWLEDGE CARDS** **(see pp. 110–111)** Use these to reflect on the kinds of knowledge that underlies your 'doing'
(ii) Standard *The ability to set up and carry out procedures to a high level of practice such that close supervision is no longer necessary*	DOPS, OP COMP and OCAPs give useful formative experience, but do not aim to give summative evidence to satisfy the standard. TA is a summative assessment that if performed rigorously attends to the standard	*In respect of the standard to be achieved,* this offers a means of uncovering, exploring and developing the drivers of our actions. This creates the evidence of the level of supervision needed by the individual doctor and clarifies any remedial needs

Element of practice to be learnt and assessed, and standard to be aimed for	Assessment methods found in national curricula (mainly 'Tools of the Trade') and the quality of evidence they produce	Means of gaining evidence of the invisible aspects of practice and how the quality of evidence available relates to the standard to be achieved
4. Clinical thinking that the practitioner engages in		
(i) Definition **The ability to engage successfully in:** • **framing the case** • **clinical reasoning** • **clinical solutions** • **deliberation** • **practical wisdom** • **using personal professional judgement**	**CASE-BASED DISCUSSION**	**THE CLINICAL THINKING PATHWAY (see pp. 125 and 132) (starting from the top down and from the bottom up)**
(ii) Standard *The ability to be focused and fluent about each given case in respect of all the aspects listed above*	C-bD offers a truncated and generalized version of the thinking that has happened, and does not require a rigorous unearthing of all the implicit and tacit thinking that has occurred	*In respect of the standard to be achieved, this offers practice in bringing together all that conduces to fluent clinical thinking.* It offers ways of collecting the evidence of the quality of thinking about given cases and across cases. It therefore enables clear evidence to be provided of whether the doctor has reached the standard and makes clear the basis for determining any remedial work necessary

5. The ability to formulate sound professional judgements and to engage in wise practice

	There is no means of assessing this in depth	Use the following to help reflection:
(i) Definition The ability to select from a range of possible judgements a high-quality professional judgement		**THE TABLE OF PROFESSIONAL JUDGEMENTS** (see pp. 152–3)
(ii) Standard *Consistency of sound professional judgement that is the best for each individual patient and the capacity to defend/argue for, implement, and lead consequent actions*	No reliable evidence of how these judgements are reached (the actions could be the result of either sound clinical thinking or good luck), and there will be no conclusive evidence of which of these is the case	*In respect of the standard to be achieved,* this offers ways of thinking about the quality of the decision made *and revealing the thinking process that lay behind it.* It therefore enables clear evidence to be provided of whether the doctor has reached the standard and makes clear the basis for determining any remedial work necessary

6. The ability to establish a sound therapeutic relationship with the patient and engage in holistic medical practice

	CASE-BASED DISCUSSION	Use the following to help reflection:
(i) Definition A wise doctor is one who can harness consideration of all the elements of practice in the best interests of each patient and establish a restorative and healing relationship with them (irrespective of the ability to cure) that enriches both doctor and patient	Only in respect of the *tone*, which is not documented in the form	**THE BEDSIDE PICTURE** (see p. 162) **ALL THE 'INVISIBLES'** Attend further to personal statement of professional philosophy

Element of practice to be learnt and assessed, and standard to be aimed for	Assessment methods found in national curricula (mainly 'Tools of the Trade') and the quality of evidence they produce	Means of gaining evidence of the invisible aspects of practice and how the quality of evidence available relates to the standard to be achieved
(ii) Standard *Consistency of the therapeutic relationship, meaning that it is established with every patient as far as is possible and not just with those with whom it is easy to work*	The 'tone' of the case discussed in C-bD is rarely considered and can be 'put on' rather than genuine; unless the doctor is asked to discuss the therapeutic relationship, it can only be glimpsed occasionally in everyday practice	*In respect of the standard to be achieved,* this offers ways of thinking about the quality of each doctor/patient relationship as well as the conduct, decisions made *and the* thinking process that lay behind them. It therefore enables all the evidence necessary to be provided in respect of the ability to establish consistently sound therapeutic relationships

7. The ability to work reflectively in the socially and clinically complex practice setting and extend and deepen a holistic vision of clinical practice

(i) Definition The ability to reflect during practice as well as afterwards, and to notice and be able to explore the ever-wider and deeper aspects of practice (both the social and the clinical) that become evident with increasing experience	**REQUIRED IN THE PORTFOLIO** (but no indication of how it can be assessed)	Use the following to reflect on complex cases and experiences: **ALL THE INVISIBLES** Use the following to explore and investigate and thus refine practice: **HUMANISTIC INVESTIGATIVE PROCESSES**

(ii) Standard
Consistency of overall development

No criteria have been developed for how to assess the portfolio, and thus there is no concrete evidence for either the learner or future teachers of whether or not a learner's progress is sound and consistent

In respect of the standard to be achieved, this offers the means of providing evidence of overall progress, indicates ways of developing practice and lays the foundation for a gradual emancipation from teachers

References

Abbot H Porter (2002) *The Cambridge Introduction to Narrative*. Cambridge: Cambridge University Press.

Bauman Z (2000) *Liquid Modernity*. Cambridge: Polity Press.

Bauman Z (2005) The liquid modern challenges to education. In: Robinson S, Katulushi C, eds. *Values in Higher Education*. Leeds: Aureus/University of Leeds.

Berger J, Mohr J (1967) *A Fortunate Man: The Story of a Country Doctor*. Harmondsworth: Penguin Press.

Brigley S, Golby M, Robbé I (2004) The educational evaluation of the General Professional Practice of Surgery (GPPS). *Ann R Coll Surg Engl* **86**: 385–7.

Broadfoot P (1996) Educational assessment: the myth of measurement. Inaugural Lecture given at the University of Bristol on 25 October 1993. In: Woods P, ed. *Contemporary Issues on Teaching and Learning*. London: Routledge/Open University: pp. 203–33.

Campbell A (1984) *Moderated Love: A Theology of Professional Care*. London: SPCK.

Carr D (1993) Questions of competence. *Br J Educ Studi* **41**: 253–71.

Carr W (1995) *For Education: Towards Critical Educational Inquiry*. Buckingham: Open University Press.

Chang RW, Bordage G, Connell KJ (1998) The importance of early problem representation during case presentations. *Acad Med* **73**(10 Suppl): 109–11.

Claxton G (2000) The anatomy of intuition. In: Atkinson P, Claxton G, eds. *The Intuitive Practitioner: On the Advantages of Not Always Knowing What One is Doing*. Buckingham: Open University Press.

Cox K (1999) *Doctor and Patient: Exploring Clinical Thinking*. Sydney: University of New South Wales Press.

Davies C (1998) Care and the transformation of professionalism. In: Knijn T, Sevenhuijsen S, eds. *Care, Citizenship and Social Cohesion*. Utrecht: Netherlands School of Social and Economic Policy Research.

Davies C, Findlay L, Bullman A, eds. (2000) *Changing Practice in Health and Social Care*. London: Open University/Sage Publications: 343–54.

de Cossart L, Fish D (2002) Membership of a profession. Part Two: The nature of professional knowledge in medical practice. *Mersey Deanery Newsletter* **14**(2). Liverpool: Mersey Deanery.

de Cossart L, Fish D (2005) *Cultivating a Thinking Surgeon: New Perspectives on Clinical Teaching, Learning and Assessment*. Shrewsbury: tfm Publications.

de Cossart L, Fish D (2006) Thinking outside the (tick) box: Rescuing professionalism and professional judgement. *Med Educ* **40**: 403–4.

Eraut M, du Boulay B (2000) *Developing the Attributes of Medical Professional Judgement and Competence*. Brighton: University of Sussex: (http://www.cogs.susx.ac.uk/users/bend/doh/reporthmtl.hmtl).

Fish D (1998) *Appreciating Practice in the Caring Professions: Refocusing Professional Development and Practitioner Research*. Oxford: Butterworth Heinemann.

Fish D, Coles C, eds. (1998) *Developing Professional Judgement in Health Care: Learning through the critical Appreciation of Practice*. Oxford: Butterworth Heinemann.

Fish D, Coles C (2005) *Medical Education: Developing A Curriculum for Practice*. Maidenhead: Open University Press.

Fish D, Higgs J (2007) The context of clinical decision-making in the Twenty First Century. In: Higgs J, Jones M, Loftus S, Christensen N, eds. *Clinical Reasoning in the Health Professions*, 3rd edn. Edinburgh: Elsevier.

Fish D, Twinn S (1997) *Quality Clinical Supervision in the Health Care Professions: Principled Approaches to Practice*. Oxford: Butterworth Heinemann.

Freidson E (1994) *Professionalism Reborn: Theory, Prophecy and Policy*. Oxford: Polity Press.

Freidson E (2001) *Professionalism: the Third Way*. Oxford: Polity Press.

Gawande A (2001) *Complications: A Surgeon's Notes on an Imperfect Science*. London: Profile Books.

General Medical Council (2006) *Good Medical Practice*. London: General Medical Council.

Golby M (1993) Educational research. In: *Educational Research: Trick or Treat?* Exeter Society for Curriculum Studies **15**(3): 5–8.

Golby M, Parrott A (1999) *Educational Research and Educational Practice*. Exeter: Fair Way Press.

Grant J, Marsden P (1988) Primary knowledge, medical education and consultant expertise: *Med Educ* **22**: 173–9.

Greenhalgh T, Hurwitz B (1998a) Why study narrative? In: Greenhalgh T, Hurwitz B, eds. *Narrative Based Medicine: Dialogue and Discourse in Clinical Practice*. London: BMJ Books.

Greenhalgh T, Hurwitz B, eds. (1998b) *Narrative Based Medicine: Dialogue and Discourse in Clinical Practice.* London: BMJ Books.

Heath I (1995) *The Mystery of General Practice.* London: Nuffield Provincial Hospitals Trust.

Heath I (1998) Following the story: continuity of care in general practice. In: Greenhalgh T, Hurwitz B, eds. *Narrative Based Medicine: Dialogue and Discourse in Clinical Practice.* London: BMJ Books.

Higgs J, Andressen A, Fish D (2004) Practice knowledge – its nature, sources and contexts. In: Higgs J, Richardson B, Abrandt Dahlgren M, eds. *Developing Practice Knowledge for Health Professionals.* Oxford: Butterworth Heinemann.

Higgs J, Fish D, Rothwell R (2007) Knowledge generation and clinical reasoning in practice. In: Higgs J, Jones M, Loftus S, Christensen N, eds. *Clinical Reasoning in the Health Professions*, 3rd edn. Edinburgh: Elsevier.

Holmes J (1998) Narrative in psychotherapy. In: Greenhalgh T, Hurwitz B, eds. *Narrative Based Medicine: Dialogue and Discourse in Clinical Practice.* London: BMJ Books.

Hurwitz, B (1998) The wounded storyteller: narrative strands in medical negligence. In: Greenhalgh T, Hurwitz B, eds. *Narrative Based Medicine: Dialogue and Discourse in Clinical Practice.* London: BMJ Books.

Johnson AG (1990) *Pathways in Medical Ethics.* London: Edward Arnold.

Joyce J (1998) A painful case. In: *The Dubliners.* London: Penguin [originally published 1914].

Kirk RM, Cox K (2004) Decision making. In: Kirk RM, Ribbans WJ, eds. *Clinical Surgery in General*, 4th edn. London: Churchill Livingstone.

Montgomery K (2006) *How Doctors Think: Clinical Judgement and the Practice of Medicine.* Oxford: Oxford University Press.

Neuberger J (2005) *The Moral State We're In: A Manifesto For a 21st Century Society.* London: HarperCollins.

O'Neill O (2002) *A Question of Trust (The 2002 Reith Lectures).* Cambridge: Cambridge University Press.

Passmore J (1998) *The Philosophy of Teaching.* London: Duckworth.

Pereira Grey D (2002) Deprofessionalising doctors? *BMJ* **324**: 627–8.

RCP (2005) *Doctors in Society, Medical Professionalism in a Changing World: Report of a Working Party.* London: Royal College of Physicians.

Ryle G (1949) *The Concept of Mind.* Harmondsworth: Penguin.

Sackett DL, Richardson S, Rosenburg W, Haynes RB (1997) *Evidence-Based Medicine: How to Practise and Teach It.* Edinburgh: Churchill Livingstone.

Saks M (1998) Professionalism and health care. In: Taylor S, Field D, eds. *Sociological Perspectives on Health, Illness and Health Care.* Oxford: Blackwell Science.

Schön D (1987a) *Educating the Reflective Practitioner.* New York: Jossey Bass.

Schön D (1987b) Changing patterns of enquiry in work and living (the Thomas Cubitt Lecture). *J R Soc Art* **6357**: 26–33.

Schmidt HG, Boshuizen HPA, Norman GR (1992) Reflection on the nature of expertise in Medicine. In: Keravnou E, ed. *Deep Models of Medical Knowledge Engineering*: Amsterdam: Elsevier: 231–48.

Southern G, Braithwaite J (1998) The end of professionalism? In: *Social Science and Medicine* **46**(1): 23–28. (Also, abridged, in: Davies C, Findlay L, Bullman A, eds. (2000) *Changing Practice in Health and Social Care*. London: Open University/Sage Publications: 300–7.)

Stenhouse L (1975) *An Introduction to Curriculum Research and Development*. London: Heinemann.

Wilkes R (1981) *Social Work with Undervalued Groups*. London: Tavistock.

Index